Healthy Runner's Handbook

Lyle J. Micheli, MD
Former President—American College of Sports Medicine

with Mark Jenkins

Human Kinetics

Library of Congress Cataloging-in-Publication Data

Micheli, Lyle J., 1940-
    Healthy runner's handbook / Lyle J. Micheli ; with Mark Jenkins.
        p.   cm.
    Includes index.
    ISBN 0-88011-524-6
    1. Running injuries--Prevention--Handbooks, manuals, etc.
    I. Jenkins, Mark, 1962-   . II. Title.
    RC1220.R8M53   1996
    613.7'172--dc20   95-26222
                                                                              CIP

ISBN: 0-88011-524-6

Developmental Editor: Kirby Mittelmeier; **Assistant Editor:** Chad Johnson; **Editorial Assistant:** Amy Carnes; **Copyeditor:** Bob Replinger; **Proofreader:** Pam Johnson; **Indexer:** Joan Griffitts; **Typesetters:** Angela K. Snyder and Kathy Fuoss; **Text Designer:** Judy Henderson; **Layout Artist:** Angela K. Snyder; **Photo Editor:** Boyd LaFoon; **Cover Designer:** Stuart Cartwright; **Photographer (cover):** F-Stock/David Stoecklein; **Illustrators:** Keith Blomberg and Jennifer Delmotte; **Printer:** United Graphics

Human Kinetics books are available at special discounts for bulk purchase. Special editions or book excerpts also can be created to specification. For details, contact the Special Sales Manager at Human Kinetics.

Printed in the United States of America   10   9   8   7   6   5   4   3   2   1

Human Kinetics
Web site: http://www.humankinetics.com/

United States: Human Kinetics
P.O. Box 5076
Champaign, IL 61825-5076
1-800-747-4457
e-mail: humank@hkusa.com

Canada: Human Kinetics, Box 24040
Windsor, ON N8Y 4Y9
1-800-465-7301 (in Canada only)
e-mail: humank@hkcanada.com

Europe: Human Kinetics, P.O. Box IW14
Leeds LS16 6TR, United Kingdom
(44) 1132 781708
e-mail: humank@hkeurope.com

Australia: Human Kinetics
57A Price Avenue
Lower Mitcham, South Australia 5062
(08) 277 1555
e-mail: humank@hkaustralia.com

New Zealand: Human Kinetics
P.O. Box 105-231, Auckland 1
(09) 523 3462
e-mail: humank@hknewz.com

In this year, which marks the 100th anniversary of the Boston Marathon, we are pleased to dedicate this book to the thousands of volunteers and runners from Massachusetts and around the world who have helped to make our marathon one of the world's premier running events.

Contents

Preface

No sport fosters more personal commitment and loyalty to an activity than running. Enthusiasm for this fitness activity is so overwhelming that for millions of runners, it is not just a sport but a way of life. This zeal drives many runners to push their bodies to new physical limits. The result, all too often, is overuse injury. *Running* magazine estimates that 80 percent of runners develop overuse injuries, and that may be a conservative figure.

Along with the running boom and its high injury rate came a new breed of sports doctor—a physician who attempts not just to cure the condition, but who also seeks to discover the underlying causes of the problem and ensure the injury does not recur. Because so many runners need physical attention, much of the work of sports doctors has focused on preventing and treating their ailments. This focus on running has helped the medical community make great strides in the understanding, prevention, treatment, and rehabilitation of the overuse injuries runners incur.

The *Healthy Runner's Handbook* draws upon this latest sports medicine information and describes the most modern techniques for diagnosing, caring for, and rehabilitating injuries most common to runners. But more important, this book reveals the underlying factors that cause overuse running injuries, and provides easy-to-follow prescriptions that will allow you and other runners to continue participating safely and successfully in your favorite sport.

Acknowledgments

Several people deserve recognition for the role they played in making this book possible.

My thanks to my co-author Mark Jenkins for taking the cutting-edge sports science research findings I provided him and turning them into material that can be utilized by "regular athletes." My personal assistant Julie Power's organizational skills were as always invaluable in helping me coordinate a project of this magnitude. Kirby Mittelmeier, the book's developmental editor at Human Kinetics, did a magnificent job—first with his fat red pen and then his fine tooth comb—in turning the raw manuscript into a superb finished product. Finally, my gratitude to my wife, Ann, whose understanding I especially appreciate during those times when my always-busy schedule becomes even more hectic.

Running:
The Risks of Injury

Running is here to stay. It is impossible to ignore the legions of men and women—young and old—who continue to pound along city streets, country roads, and municipal parks. Surveys show that more than 26 million adults run regularly in the U.S. alone.

Despite the growing popularity of rival fitness forms such as aerobic dance, stairclimbing and cross-country skiing simulators, mountain biking, and in-line skating, running remains a perennial favorite. The appeal of running is obvious: almost everyone can do it; it can be done almost anywhere and at any time; and it is inexpensive. Every year it attracts growing numbers of new participants drawn to its health benefits and unique advantages.

Like most health fitness activities, running has an unfortunate downside: injuries. Most runners at one time or another succumb to a running-related ailment that puts them out of action, sometimes permanently. Plagued by sore knees, aching calves, and tender Achilles tendons, many runners reluctantly hang up their sneakers. The injuries experienced by runners are not the ordinary acute strains, sprains, bruises, and breaks traditionally seen in sports. Instead, the concern of many runners is a relatively new category of injury: overuse injuries.

Sometimes called chronic injuries, these conditions are not caused by a single trauma, but by recurrent stress to an area of the body. Runners experience this recurrent stress in the lower extremities. Given the frequency with which overuse injuries afflict runners, people began to ask: Is it possible to run without becoming injured?

The sports medicine profession, rising to the challenge, has found new ways to manage overuse injuries. By establishing the primary causes of these injuries, known as *risk factors*, and taking steps to address them, sports doctors have learned how to diagnose, treat, and rehabilitate these conditions, and perhaps most important, have discovered how they can be prevented.

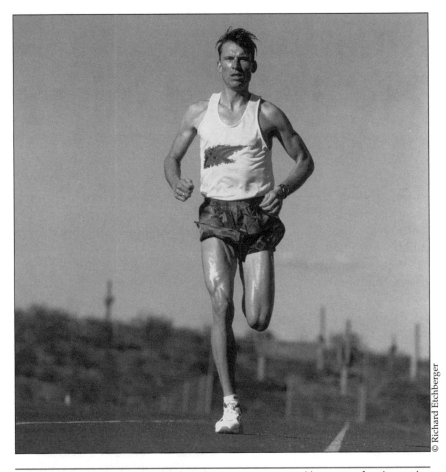

Running without injury is possible by taking precautions and becoming familiar with self-management techniques.

The response, then, to whether it is possible to run without becoming injured, is yes, so long as the runner takes the necessary precautions. Prevention is always better than cure, but runners who do become injured can avoid long-term absences from running by familiarizing themselves with the most effective ways to self-manage their conditions,

which include accurate diagnosis and efficacious treatment and rehabilitation.

Overuse Injuries and Risk Factors

When overuse injuries in running began to be perceived as inevitable, a
backlash occurred. Unlike acute injuries, which were usually the result
of accidents, overuse injuries appeared to be caused by runners doing
exactly what they were supposed to do, and therefore overuse injuries
were presumed the rule in running, not the exception.

After studying millions of overuse injuries, however, sports medicine
concluded that overuse injuries are not an inevitable by-product of running. Sports doctors have identified specific causes of overuse injury,
which are preventable. These risk factors are either *intrinsic* or *extrinsic*.

Intrinsic risk factors include

- previous injury,
- poor conditioning and muscle imbalances,
- anatomical abnormalities,
- incorrect technique, and
- nutritional abuse, which in conjunction with an intensive running
  schedule may cause stress fractures.

Extrinsic risk factors include

- training errors, including abrupt increases in intensity, duration, or
  frequency of training,
- inappropriate workout structure, and
- improper footwear.

It is not possible to overemphasize the importance of these risk factors. By addressing them, runners can drastically reduce the chance of
overuse injury. Risk factors are the key not only to prevention, but also
to diagnosis, treatment, and rehabilitation. They lie at the heart of why
some runners sustain overuse injuries, while others do not. An understanding of all the risk factors associated with overuse running injuries
is a crucial first step toward taking a comprehensive approach to running injury management.

Intrinsic Risk Factors

Of the risk factors associated with overuse running injuries, the ones
most frequently responsible for causing injuries are intrinsic: previous

injury, poor conditioning and muscle imbalances, anatomical abnor-malities, and incorrect technique. In addition, nutritional abuse can play a role in injuries suffered by female athletes.

Previous Injury

The most reliable predictor of injury is previous injury. Most runners who become injured are destined to reinjure themselves. Unless the runner does rehabilitation, tissues weakened by injury do not fully re-gain their strength, which puts them at risk of being damaged again. Furthermore, the scar tissue created by soft tissue damage makes the muscle less supple and therefore susceptible to another injury. After an injury, the runner must do exercises to restore strength and flexibility to the tissues. Athletes who do not do specific exercises after sustaining a joint injury—especially of the knee—are almost certain to reinjure the joint.

Proper rehabilitation may break the injury and reinjury cycle, but

The Musculoskeletal System

The foundation of the body is the musculoskeletal system, which is made up of muscles, bones, joints, and their associated tissues. These are the areas most often injured in sports.

Bones

Bones make up the skeleton, which is the body's framework. The skeleton has two main functions:

- Supporting the body
- Protecting important organs

Muscles

Muscles move the bones by shortening and lengthening in re-sponse to signals from the brain. The major muscle groups are the rotator cuff in the shoulder, quadriceps in the front of the thigh, hamstrings behind the thigh, biceps in front of the upper arm, triceps behind the upper arm, and the calf muscles behind the lower leg.

(continued)

Joints

Joints, where the bones meet, are the structures that enable the body to move. The shapes of the ends of the bones where they meet determine the directions in which they are able to move. Major joints include the shoulder, elbow, wrist, hip, knee, and ankle. Joints are made up of ligaments, tendons, cartilage, and bursae.

Ligaments

Ligaments hold the bones together at the joints. They are flexible but not elastic. For that reason, ligament sprains are among the most common sports injuries.

Cartilage

Cartilage is the gristly tissue found at the ends of bones. It helps absorb the impact and friction of bones bumping and rubbing against each other. It is sometimes known as joint cartilage or articular cartilage. A type of cartilage found in about 10 percent of joints is meniscus—a flat, crescent-shaped piece of cartilage that stabilizes the joint, absorbs shock, and disperses lubrication known as synovial fluid.

Bursae

Bursae are small pouches of fluid located in parts of the body where friction and stress occur. They are found between bones, muscles, tendons, and other tissues. The job of a bursa is to reduce friction between different tissue types, and protect the underlying tissue from impact.

Tendons

Tendons are the tough, narrow ends of muscles that connect muscles to bones. Like ligaments, tendons are flexible but not elastic.

only when the program emphasizes return to full function, not just symptom relief. For general rehabilitation guidelines regarding overuse injuries, see chapters 2 and 3; for specific rehabilitation approaches to individual injuries, see chapters 4 through 9.

Poor Conditioning and Muscle Imbalances

A person whose sole form of exercise is running often develops imbalances in muscle strength and flexibility. The consequence of these imbalances is threefold. First, they can cause stresses to the underlying tissues; second, they can pull certain parts of the anatomy out of alignment; and third, they may interfere with proper running form. All three can lead to overuse injuries.

Stresses Caused by Muscle Imbalances

Tight muscles may be responsible for any number of overuse running injuries. Excessive tightness in the musculature on the outside of the thigh (iliotibial band) can cause pressure on the underlying structures, leading to overuse injuries around the outside of the knee (iliotibial band friction syndrome) and the outer side of the hip (trochanteric bursitis). Tight muscles and tendons in back of the lower leg (gastrosoleus/Achilles tendon unit) can cause Achilles tendinitis, an inflammation of the thick cord of tissue that connects the calf muscles to the back of the heel, and plantar fasciitis, an inflammation of the connective tissue underneath the foot that connects the toes to the heel (plantar fascia).

Malalignments Caused by Muscle Imbalances

The most frequent sites of malalignments caused by muscle imbalances are the back and knee.

Measuring Relative Leg Strength

The relative strength between the quadriceps and hamstrings can be measured using strength training machines found at most health clubs. The leg extension machine measures the strength of the quadriceps; the leg curl machine measures the strength of the hamstrings. The strength ratio between the quadriceps and hamstrings should be no less than 3:2 in favor of the quadriceps, or problems may occur. For example, a runner who can lift 80 pounds with his or her hamstrings using the leg curl machine should be able to lift at least 120 pounds with his or her quadriceps using the leg extension machine.

Lower back pain is common in runners. Often it is caused by tightness in the muscles in front of the hip (psoas) and behind the thigh (hamstrings) relative to the stomach muscles (abdominals) and the muscles in front of the thigh (quadriceps). Such an imbalance can cause a postural abnormality called "swayback" or lordosis, in which there is excessive front-to-back curve in the lower spine. This in turn predisposes the runner to serious overuse injuries of the lower back such as herniated disk and spondylolysis.

Kneecap pain is another frequent complaint in runners. The most common kneecap problem is patellofemoral pain syndrome, which is usually caused by the kneecap (patella) tracking improperly in its groove on the thighbone. Often, this problem is caused by the tightness and strength of the muscles in back of the thigh (hamstrings) relative to the muscles in front of the thigh (quadriceps). In such circumstances, the quadriceps cannot maintain the proper straight-ahead alignment of the lower and upper leg when the person runs; as a result, the lower leg "spins out" during the running cycle, which in turn causes excessive stress to the outer side of the kneecap.

Muscle Imbalances and Overuse Running Injuries

Muscle imbalance	Possible injury consequence if subjected to repetitive stress of running
Tightness in musculature running down outer side of thigh (iliotibial band)	Iliotibial band friction syndrome
Tightness in muscle in back of lower leg (Achilles tendons and calf muscles)	Achilles tendinitis
Tightness in muscles in front of the hip (psoas) and behind the thigh (hamstrings) compared to stomach muscles (abdominals) and front of thigh muscles (quadriceps)	"Swayback" (lordosis), which may cause severe back problems such as herniated disk or spondylolysis

(continued)

Muscle imbalance	Possible injury consequence if subjected to repetitive stress of running
Tight, strong muscles in back the thigh (hamstrings) relative to muscles in front of the thigh (quadriceps)	Kneecap pain on outer sideof
Tight, strong outer thigh muscles (vastus lateralis) relative to inner thigh muscles (vastus medialis)	Kneecap pain

Another related cause of kneecap pain is an imbalance between the muscles in the inner and outer sides of the quadriceps, the vastus medialis and vastus lateralis, respectively. Frequently, the outer thigh muscles are tighter and stronger than the ones on the inner thigh. Because these muscles attach to either side of the kneecap, tighter and stronger outer thigh muscles can pull the kneecap to the outside with each step when running, a tracking problem that may result in chronic kneecap pain.

Foot Strike Problems Caused by Muscle Imbalances

The third problem associated with muscle imbalances is their effect on the biomechanics of running, or more simply, running form.

Running causes tightness in certain areas, notably the psoas muscles in front of the hip, the hamstring muscles in back of the thigh, and the gastro-soleus/Achilles tendon unit in back of the lower leg.

Runners with this pattern of tightness tend to have a much briefer-than-normal foot strike; because their muscles are so tight they cannot perform the optimal relaxed heel-to-toe foot strike. Their feet spend less time on the ground with each step and thus absorb more stress every time they hit the ground. Although the time differential may seem very minor, when one considers the runner may take 10,000 steps every hour, the consequences may be dramatic.

Self-Test for Muscle Imbalances

Muscles that are relatively tight compared to their opposing muscles can cause serious problems in runners. The muscle groups that can cause the most problems if they are excessively tight include the hip flexors, hamstrings, and calves/Achilles tendons. The following are ways to test if you have tightness in any of these muscle groups.

Hip flexors

Lie on your back. Draw both your knees to your chest with your hands. Release your right knee, continuing to hold your left knee tight to your chest. Keeping the knee of your right leg straight, try to lay it flat on the floor. Repeat with the left leg. If you cannot do this with either side, you have excessively tight hip flexor muscles. Refer to the section on stretching for exercises to overcome this specific tightness.

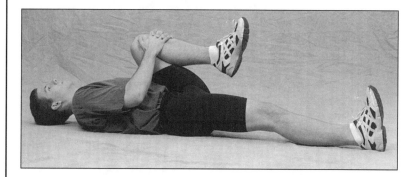

Hamstrings

Begin by lying beside a wall. Bend knees, then swing around so your body is at a right angle to the wall. Raise both legs, and, *keeping knees straight*, gently try to move your buttocks as close as

(continued)

possible to the wall. If, with your knees straight, you cannot get your buttocks closer than eight inches to the wall, then you have excessively tight hamstring muscles. Refer to the section on stretching for exercises to overcome this specific tightness.

Calves/Achilles tendons

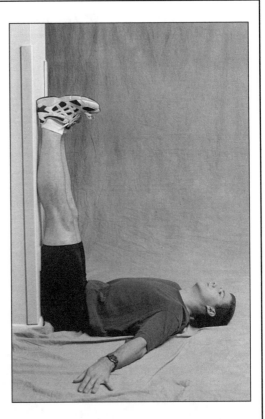

Sit on the floor, right leg out straight, left leg tucked in. Reach forward and grasp the toes of your right foot, and gently pull toward you. If you cannot get the bottom of your foot to form a right angle with the floor, you have tight calves and Achilles tendons. Refer to the section on stretching

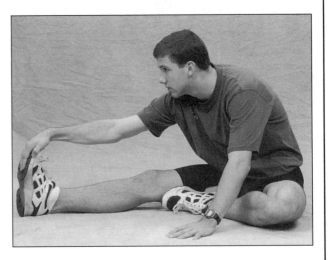

for exercises to overcome this specific tightness.

Anatomical Abnormalities

One of the most common reasons some athletes sustain overuse injuries while others do not is they have anatomical abnormalities that place additional stress on the surrounding structures. In daily activities, these anatomical abnormalities do not cause problems, but when they are subjected to the repetitive stresses of running, overuse injuries may occur. The seven most common anatomical abnormalities of the lower extremities are flat feet, feet that excessively *pronate* (roll inward when the athlete runs), high arches, turned-in thigh bones (femoral anteversion), knock knees, bow legs, and unequal leg length.

Flat Feet and Excessive Pronation

Some people have naturally flat feet that excessively turn inward (pronate) when they run. A certain amount of natural pronation occurs with each step. Excessive pronation, however, can be harmful. It causes increased stress throughout the lower extremities. In such cases, overuse injuries may occur. In the foot itself, the most common over-

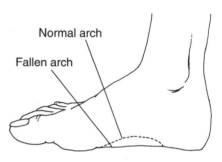

use injuries associated with flat feet and feet that excessively pronate are stress fractures and posterior tibial tendinitis.

Flat feet and feet that excessively pronate not only cause problems in the foot, but also may affect the entire lower extremities, including the knee and hip. Both these conditions cause inward rotation of the legs.

Problems in the lower extremities above the feet caused in part by flat feet or feet that excessively pronate are kneecap pain, compartment syndrome in the lower leg, and trochanteric bursitis in the hip.

High Arches

High arches, or "claw foot" as this condition is sometimes known, makes the foot inflexible. The rigidity of this kind of foot makes it susceptible to overuse injuries. It also results in overuse injuries in the lower leg because its inflexibility transmits force to the structures above.

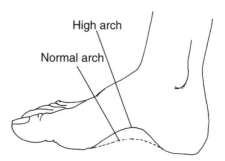

Athletes with high arches are susceptible to plantar fasciitis (heel spurs), Achilles tendinitis, and stress fractures in the foot, lower leg, upper thigh, and pelvis.

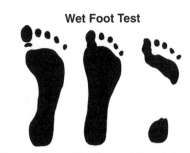

Wet Foot Test

Normal foot   Flat foot   High arches

A person with high arches may also develop a "hammer toe" in which the second toe buckles and cannot be straightened. A high arch may cause the big toe to slide under the second toe when the athlete runs, causing the hammer toe condition to develop.

A quick way to check your arch is the wet foot test.

Turned-In Thigh Bones (Femoral Anteversion)

Some people have thigh bones that turn inward. This is caused by abnormal hip joints. When this condition exists, the kneecaps face slightly inward. This can cause tracking problems in the kneecap, which is a common cause of patellofemoral pain syndrome, a very common overuse condition.

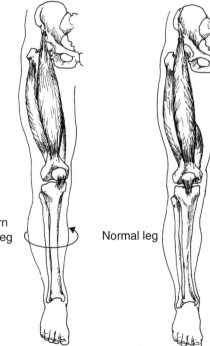

Inward turn of lower leg

Normal leg

Knock Knees

Knock knees create serious problems for the knee joints. Excessive inward angling at the point where the thigh and lower leg meet (*Q angle*) causes the runner's weight to be borne on the inside of the knee. A Q angle greater than 10 degrees in men and 15 degrees in women is said to predispose that person to knee problems if he or she participates in a rigorous running regimen. Knock knees are a common cause of patellofemoral pain syndrome, the most common diagnosis seen in sports clinics.

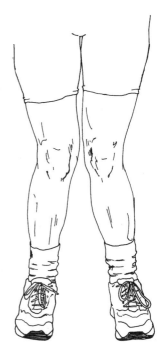

Bow Legs

Bow legs are the opposite of knock knees—they bend outward instead of angling inward. Athletes with bow legs are at risk of sustaining problems on the outer side of the knee, especially iliotibial band friction syndrome. Having bowed legs creates a longer distance over which the iliotibial band must stretch, making it tighter over the outer side of the knee joint where the symptoms develop. Many athletes with bow legs, however, participate in distance running without any problems.

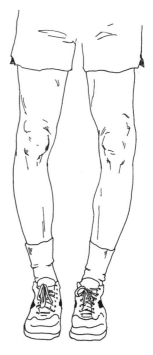

Unequal Leg Length

It is not uncommon for people to have one leg longer than the other. This can create problems, especially in the longer leg. For instance, in the longer leg the iliotibial band (the thick swathe of tissue that runs down the side of the leg from the hip to just below the knee) must stretch over a longer distance, which may cause inflammation of this

Anatomical Abnormalities and Overuse Running Injuries

Anatomical abnormality	Possible injury consequence if subjected to repetitive stress of running
Flat feet or feet that excessively turn inward when the person runs	Kneecap pain, shin pain, trochanteric bursitis in the hip, stress fractures in the feet, plantar fasciitis (bone spurs), bunions, calluses, tendinitis of the inner ankle, Achilles tendinitis
High arches	Stress fractures in the feet, lower leg, upper thigh, pelvis; plantar fasciitis (heel spurs); Achilles tendinitis; tendinitis of the outer ankle
Knock knees	Kneecap pain
Bow legs	Iliotibial band friction syndrome, tendinitis of the outer ankle
Turned-in thigh bones	Kneecap pain
Unequal leg length lower	Iliotibial band friction syndrome, back pain, trochanteric bursitis in the hip

tissue where it passes over the outer side of the knee joint. Also, a person with one leg longer than the other tends to run with his or her spine curved slightly sideways. As a result, wear and tear may occur on the concave side of the spine.

Incorrect Technique

Running would seem to be a fairly straightforward activity learned in childhood, but many people run using poor technique. This may not cause problems when running short distances in daily activities, but may result in overuse injuries when those people participate in distance running.

For instance, runners who land exceedingly hard on their heels may develop stress fractures in the foot. Conversely, those who run on their tiptoes can develop tight calf muscles and Achilles tendons with the resulting problems.

Improper running technique may be associated with the tightness caused by running itself (see the earlier section "Poor Conditioning and Muscle Imbalances").

Menstrual Irregularities and Eating Disorders in Women

Female athletes tend to suffer more eating disorders than sedentary women. This is especially true for recreational athletes who engage in sports and exercise primarily for weight control.

The combination of poor eating habits and high activity level can cause a woman's fat level to drop below the level necessary for normal menstrual function. When women stop having their periods or have periods irregularly, they lose much of the estrogen necessary for the bone rebuilding that normal bodies perform on a continuous basis. This can cause premature osteoporosis, a disease that causes the bones to become thinner and more brittle, which in turn predisposes the athlete to stress fractures. Among young female athletes with menstrual irregularities, the incidence of stress fractures is almost three times normal. The most common sites of stress fractures in female athletes are the back, hip, pelvis, lower leg, and foot. For more information on this risk factor, see chapter 10, "Special Concerns for Female Runners."

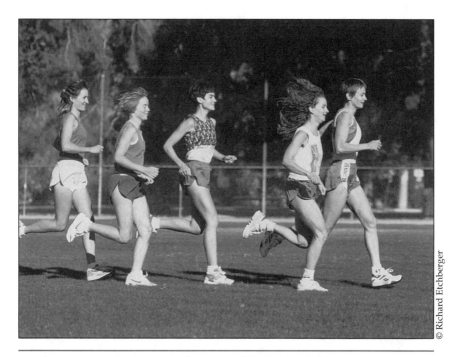

Female runners need to be especially aware of their eating habits.

Extrinsic Risk Factors

Of extrinsic risk factors contributing to running injuries, training error is by far the most common. Improper workout structure and inappropriate footwear can also play a role.

Errors in Training

Training error—usually trying to do too much too soon—is a primary cause of injury, especially overuse injury. Injuries can develop when athletes suddenly increase the *frequency, duration,* or *intensity* of their workouts.

Frequency refers to *how often* the athlete trains.

Duration refers to *how long* the athlete trains.

Intensity refers to *how hard* the athlete trains. Not only does intensity encompass factors such as how far or how fast a person jogs or how heavy a weight he or she lifts, it also refers to less obvious aspects of the exercise regimen, such as the hardness of the training surface. Joggers should know they have increased the intensity of their workout if they

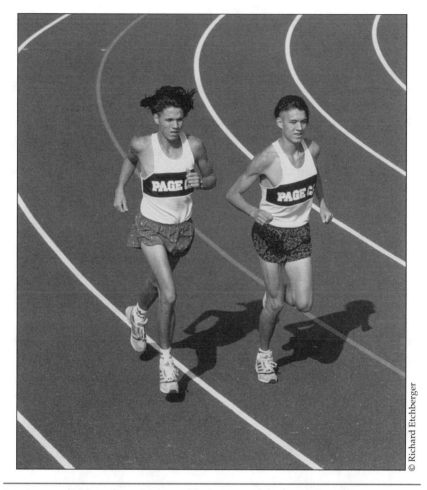

Injuries can develop when runners suddenly increase the frequency, duration, or intensity of their workouts.

switch from running on grass or clay to road running, or from running primarily on flat surfaces to running hills. Softer does not always mean less stressful; for instance, running on sand stresses the Achilles tendons and predisposes the athlete to tendinitis in that area. See "Avoid Training Errors" in chapter 2 for ways to prevent injuries caused by this risk factor.

Improper Workout Structure

A common cause of injury is the failure to prepare the body for exercise with a structured workout that includes warm-up and cool-down periods. Warming up and cooling down (sometimes called warming down) are relatively new concepts in recreational sports, but should be part of every athlete's workout routine.

Less pliable tissues in the body are more susceptible to overuse injuries: tiny tears may occur due to repetitive, low-intensity stretching of inflexible tissues. Overuse injuries of the joints can develop because the surrounding tissues are not warmed up and stretched, which restricts the joint's range of motion and may cause grinding of the cartilage against bone or cartilage against other cartilage.

The intensity and duration of the warm-up and cool-down varies with each athlete. A well-conditioned athlete probably requires a

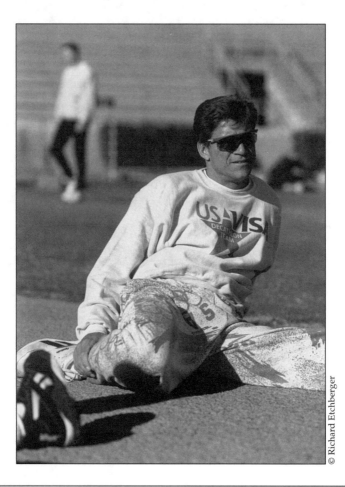

© Richard Etchberger

Cool-down stretching should be part of every athlete's workout.

longer, more intense warm-up than a less well-conditioned person to achieve optimal elevation in body temperature and heart rate.

Irrespective of the conditioning level of the athlete, every workout should include five stages: limbering up (5 minutes); stretching (5-10 minutes); warm-up (5 minutes); primary activity; and cool-down stretching (10 minutes). We look at workout structure in greater detail in chapter 2.

Using the Risk Factor Checklist to Determine Cause of Injury

Sports doctors use a checklist of risk factors to determine how runners become injured. Runners can use the same checklist.

✓ "Did I recently increase the frequency, duration, or intensity of my running regimen by more than 10 percent?" *If the answer is yes, the underlying cause of your overuse injury may be* **training error.**

✓ "Is running the only exercise I do?" "Are some of my muscles naturally not as strong or flexible as adjoining ones?" *If the answer is yes, the underlying cause of your overuse running injury may be* **imbalances in muscle strength and flexibility.**

✓ "Do I have flat feet, high arches, bow legs, knock knees, thighs that turn inward from the hip, or one leg longer than the other?" *If the answer is yes, the underlying cause of your overuse running injury may be an* **anatomical abnormality.**

✓ "Are my running shoes old or worn-out?" "Did I recently start using new running shoes?" *If the answer is yes, the underlying cause of your overuse running injury may be* **improper footwear.**

✓ "Did I neglect to structure my run to include limbering-up, stretching, a warm-up, a cool-down, and a cool-down stretch?" *If the answer is yes, the underlying cause of your overuse running injury may be an* **inappropriate workout structure.**

(continued)

✓ "Did I not fully rehabilitate a previous running injury?" *If the answer is yes, the underlying cause of your overuse running injury may be* **previous injury.**

✓ "Do I fail to engage in a strength and flexibility program related to my running program?" *If the answer is yes, the underlying cause of your overuse running injury may be* **poor conditioning.**

✓ "Do I have an unusual running style?" *If the answer is yes, the underlying cause of your injury may be* **improper running technique.**

✓ "Do I run frequently, but menstruate irregularly or not at all?" *If women answer yes, the underlying cause of your overuse running injury may be* **nutritional abuse.**

Inappropriate Footwear

Runners exert with each step a combined force of three to four times their body weight. That force is absorbed by the running surface, the shoe, and the foot and leg. The less force the limb absorbs, the less risk there is of overuse injury. That explains why it is better to train on slightly softer surfaces like clay or grass rather than on cement or asphalt, which have less "give." It also explains why shoes are the most important wardrobe item for most athletes.

Shoes are especially important for runners. The right footwear makes for an enjoyable, injury-free running experience, while the wrong footwear can cause discomfort and ailments ranging from ankle sprains to heel spurs to knee cartilage tears.

Thankfully, improvements in the last decade have contributed to a decline in many footwear-related overuse injuries. All runners should know how to select the right footwear. See pages 61-66 for more information on running shoes.

Addressing Risk Factors Associated With Overuse Running Injuries

A comprehensive program to prevent, manage, and rehabilitate running injuries by addressing each of these risk factors is discussed in the chapters that follow. Chapter 2 focuses on prevention. Chapter 3 gives general guidelines for injury diagnosis and management. In chapters 4 through 9 we take a close look at overuse injuries associated with specific parts of the body and address their contributing risk factors, symptoms, treatments, and cures. The remaining chapters discuss special concerns for women and nutrition.

Prevention of Running Injuries

Most running injuries are preventable. Runners can avoid injury by familiarizing themselves with the primary causes of running injuries, known as risk factors. The risk factors associated with running injuries are divided into those factors particular to the individual runner, intrinsic risk factors, and those associated with the sport itself, extrinsic risk factors. By addressing these risk factors, runners can greatly reduce their chances of becoming injured.

Addressing Intrinsic Risk Factors

The following sections describe the most effective ways of addressing intrinsic risk factors associated with running.

Fully Rehabilitate Previous Injuries

Rehabilitation is the process of using exercise to return to action. Runners who do not rehabilitate their injuries are unlikely to regain full function in the injured area and are much more likely to be reinjured. Indeed, the main predictor of injury is previous injury. The high incidence of injury in running and the data suggesting that reinjury is likely reinforces the importance of rehabilitation in injury management.

Rehabilitation can break a runner's injury and reinjury cycle—so long as the rehabilitation is appropriate for the injury and the program is geared toward restoring function, not just relieving the symptoms. Unfortunately, too many athletes return to action when their symptoms have abated without having addressed the underlying cause of their condition.

In the case of a serious injury or one that requires surgery, rehabilitation should be supervised by a doctor and a physical therapist. Professionally supervised rehabilitation for runners has the same goals as self-managed rehabilitation. Besides ice and heat, the rehabilitation team may employ more sophisticated therapeutic modalities such as ultrasound and electric stimulation.

Refer to chapter 3, "Diagnosis and Management of Running Injuries," for more on the general principles of rehabilitating running injuries, and chapters 4 through 9 for specific rehabilitation regimens for individual injuries.

Use Proper Technique

As seen earlier, running itself can create tightness in certain muscle groups, which may make it difficult for the runner to observe proper running form. This may in turn cause injuries. Specifically, runners with characteristic tightness in the psoas muscles in front of the hip, hamstring muscles in back of the thigh, and the gastro-soleus/Achilles tendon unit in back of the lower leg tend to have a much briefer-than-normal foot strike; because their muscles are so tight they cannot perform the optimal relaxed heel-to-toe foot strike. Their feet spend much less time on the ground than they should so they have to absorb much more stress each time they hit the ground. To restore proper running form, athletes with tightness in the previously mentioned muscle groups should engage in a flexibility program.

Some people simply use improper running technique. The following are some general guidelines on technique:

- Run in an upright position, avoiding excessive forward lean. Keep back as straight as is comfortable, and keep head up. Do not look downward at feet.
- Carry arms slightly away from the body, with elbows bent so forearms are roughly parallel to ground. Occasionally shake and relax arms to prevent tightness in shoulders.
- Land on the heel of the foot and rock forward to drive off the ball of the foot. If this is difficult, try a more flat-footed style. Running

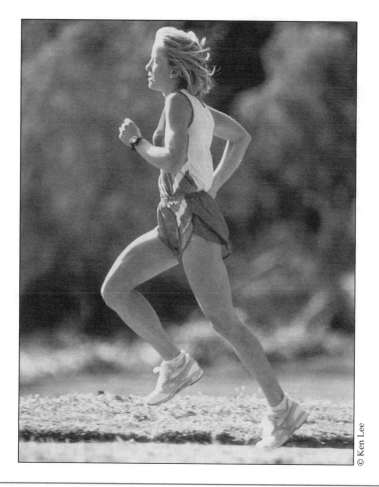

© Ken Lee

Focusing on correct running technique is a great way to help prevent overuse injuries.

on the balls of the feet will cause the runner to tire quickly and make the legs sore.
- Keep strides short. Do not force the pace by reaching for extra distance.
- Breathe deeply with mouth open.

Minimize the Effects of Anatomical Abnormalities

Anatomical abnormalities of the lower extremities are another frequent cause of overuse injury in runners. In daily activities, these anatomical abnormalities do not cause problems, but when they are subjected to the

Running and Air Pollution

Runners who train in an environment that is smog laden, carbon monoxide loaded, and ozone filled may be doing themselves more harm than good. With pollution from internal combustion engines and industrial sources now such a problem, air pollution may soon become a major health concern for athletes who exercise outdoors.

Until recently, air pollution was a problem mainly in congested urban areas, where automobile and industrial exhausts are primary offenders, or in cities nestled in mountain basins where these same pollutants are trapped by atmospheric inversions. Now, rural areas are also affected, not only by forest fires, agricultural burning, and mining operations, but by pollutants blown from cities or industrial areas.

Runners with no choice but to exercise in polluted conditions can take the following precautions to minimize health risks:

- Check air quality reports on the newspaper weather page or call the regional office of the Department of Environmental Conservation and ask for the current Pollutant Standard Index (PSI) level. Readings in the range of 100 to 199 are considered unhealthy. When pollution levels are high, exercise before 10 A.M., before ozone has the chance to build up.
- Avoid running near heavily traveled roadways. If possible, run in open, windswept areas, where pollutants are easily dispersed. To avoid the exhaust of passing vehicles, run on the upwind side of the road.
- Reduce running intensity and duration when pollution levels are high or when breathing is impaired.
- When competing in a polluted area, minimize physical activity before the event to reduce the dose of pollutants. Reduce the intensity of the warm-up before competition.
- Stop if breathing is difficult. Constricted air passages are a warning that air quality is poor.
- When pollution levels are unacceptable, train indoors. Instead of focusing on treadmill running that places a heavy demand on breathing, emphasize weight training with reduced sets and repetitions. Make use of this time to focus on flexibility, technique, and strategies specific to running.

repetitive stresses of running, overuse injuries may occur. The most common anatomical abnormalities of the lower extremities are flat feet that excessively roll inward when the athlete runs, high arches, knock knees, bow legs, turned-in thighbones (femoral anteversion), and unequal leg length. For the specific relationships between anatomical abnormalities and overuse injuries, see page 14.

Anatomical abnormalities may be the risk factor that is most difficult to overcome. For example, runners who lack rotation in the hips, particularly internal rotation, may never be able to run without a repetitive pattern of injuries. These people may have to take up a fitness activity other than running.

If you have an anatomical abnormality or suspect that you have one and you have developed an overuse injury, consult a sports doctor.

To realign the lower extremities and prevent the anatomical abnormality from creating problems, the doctor's most frequent course of action is to prescribe either shoe inserts (orthotics) or an exercise program.

Shoe inserts are often used to correct flat feet, feet that pronate (roll inward when the person runs), and high arches. If the condition is mild, the doctor may recommend an over-the-counter orthotic. OTC orthotics are most appropriate for runners with mild anatomical abnormalities. If OTC orthotics do not alleviate an overuse condition, or if the doctor deems the anatomical abnormality to be severe, the doctor may prescribe custom-made orthotics.

There are two types of custom-made orthotics—soft and rigid.

Soft orthotics are prescribed for high arches. High arches make the foot very inflexible, reducing its ability to efficiently absorb repetitive impact. Runners with high arches are thus susceptible to overuse conditions such as stress fractures, heel spurs, and Achilles tendinitis.

Soft orthotics are usually made using the weightbearing method. In this technique the athlete steps into a foam-filled box and makes an imprint of his or her feet. This imprint provides an impression of the feet from which a model of the foot is made, and a corrective orthotic can be made.

Besides providing much needed cushioning support for high arches, soft orthotics also provide impact absorption that prevents conditions such as heel spurs, plantar fasciitis, and stress fractures.

Rigid orthotics are preferable for flat feet and feet that excessively pronate. Their purpose is to restrict excessive rolling-in of the foot when running—the undesirable motion associated with flat feet. As shown in the accompanying illustration, the orthotic device in *a* helps prevent the foot's collapse into excessive pronation at foot strike (as seen in *b* without the device). Overuse injuries commonly seen in runners with feet that excessively pronate are stress fractures, posterior tibial tendinitis, and compartment syndromes of the lower leg.

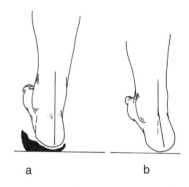

a   b

A nonweightbearing technique is used to fit rigid orthotics to the runner. Using plaster of paris, an imprint of the foot is made while the athlete is sitting or lying down with his or her legs hanging off the edge of a table. When the plaster has dried, the negative cast is filled with wet plaster to make a model of the foot from which an orthotic is designed to correct the anatomical abnormality.

Having the model of the foot made when the athlete is lying down allows a much more accurate biomechanical evaluation of the runner's foot. Because they require more skill to fit, podiatrists and orthotists usually make rigid orthotics.

Although orthotics are often prescribed to alleviate high arches, they are frequently ineffective. Sometimes static stretching of the arch may be

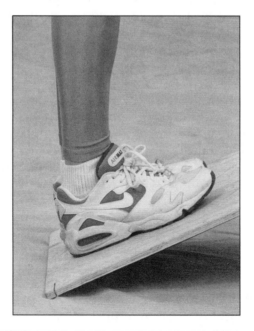

Static stretching on an inclined board may help alleviate problems caused by high arches.

of some assistance in alleviating the problem. The athlete should stand on a board inclined at a 35-degree angle, 20 to 30 seconds at a time, first with the toes facing downward, and then with the toes facing upward. When doing static stretches, the runner should point the toes inward slightly. If pain continues, the runner may not have any choice other than to take up a different sport.

Runners with bow legs are susceptible to iliotibial band friction syndrome, an inflammation of the tissue on the outer side of the knee. Having bowed legs creates a longer distance over which the iliotibial band must stretch, making it tighter over the outer side of the knee joint, where symptoms develop. To prevent this condition, runners with bowed legs should emphasize stretching the iliotibial band during their prerunning stretch.

Improve Conditioning and Correct Muscle Imbalances

When done exclusively, running tends to tighten and strengthen muscle groups in certain areas. This can cause imbalances of strength and flexibility, which may in turn lead to overuse injuries in the back, hip, knee, lower leg, and foot.

If the runner can detect an imbalance in strength or flexibility, he or she should participate in a conditioning program to redress those imbalances. Refer to pages 9-10 for a self-test to detect muscle imbalances (if

Tendon Injuries

Tendons are the tough, ropelike tissues that connect muscle to bone. They are strong but not very flexible.

In sports where repetitive movement is required, such as running, tendons become injured from frequent, low-intensity overloading.

Tendon overuse injuries are known as tendinitis. This condition refers to microtears of a tendon caused by repetitive, low-intensity overstretching. For instance, Achilles tendinitis is common in runners because of the repetitive stretching of the heel cord. Other tendon injuries seen in runners are iliotibial band syndrome (knee) and patellar tendinitis (knee).

(continued)

Like many overuse injuries, tendinitis is often ignored because the symptoms develop slowly. Few sports injuries, however, are as difficult to treat as tendinitis. Because of poor blood supply, healing is very slow. For this reason, it is crucial that runners who develop tendinitis treat the condition early to avoid extended lay-offs from sports and long-term dysfunction.

Preventing tendinitis

Prevent tendinitis from developing in the first place by following these guidelines:

- Have a presports physical to (1) rule out natural tendon tightness that causes microtears in the tendon fibers due to normal stretching during physical activity and (2) rule out imbalances in strength or flexibility between any tendons and their adjoining muscles, or between tendons on one side of a muscle-tendon unit and tendons on the opposing side.
- Engage in a conditioning program to develop strength and flexibility in the muscle-tendon units so they are not as vulnerable to microtears in the tendon fibers due to normal stretching during physical activity.
- Perform a proper warm-up and cool-down before physical activity to prepare the tendon fibers for the normal stretching of exercise.
- Wear appropriate footwear to reduce or eliminate over-stretching of the Achilles tendon during exercise.
- Observe a progressive training regimen to minimize rapid increases in exercise frequency, duration, or intensity that can overstress the tendon.

Prevent mild tendinitis from becoming a chronic condition by following these guidelines:

- Cease running.
- Use the RICE prescription.
- Take acetaminophen or ibuprofen as label-directed.
- Do not return to running until there is absolutely no localized tenderness or pain when using the muscle-tendon unit.

(continued)

- Gradually return to running when the symptoms are gone.
- Seek medical attention if the condition persists for more than two weeks, despite conservative self-treatment.

Prevent a chronic tendinitis condition from becoming permanently dysfunctional by following these guidelines:

- Withdraw immediately from running.
- Use the RICE prescription.
- Take acetaminophen or ibuprofen as label-directed.
- Seek expert medical attention as soon as possible.
- Carefully follow the rehabilitation program and do not return to running until cleared by the doctor and the physical therapist.
- Gradually return to running.

in doubt, consult a sports doctor to determine whether you have imbalances in muscle strength or flexibility, and what steps to take to overcome the problems they are causing, if any).

Flexibility Training

The most frequently asked questions concerning a flexibility program involve how often it is done (frequency), how hard it is done (intensity), and how long it is done (duration).

Frequency: The runner should stretch daily. If there is tightness in a particular area (the hamstrings, for example), the runner should exercise that area twice a day.

Intensity: Stretch to the point of tension, known as the action point. By not overstretching the muscle, runners can relax while they are stretching and thus hold each position longer.

Duration: The maximum benefit comes from holding the stretch for a full 60 seconds. This is because it may take from 20 to 40 seconds for the muscles to fully relax. By holding the stretch for 60 seconds, the athlete knows that the tight muscles, tendons, and ligaments are being stretched slowly, with a minimal chance of injury. Stretches between 10 and 30 seconds, however, can provide benefits. If the athlete is unable to hold a position for the specified time because he or she becomes tired, that is acceptable. He or she can rest, or, where appropriate, switch to the other limb. Athletes should perform the stretch as many times as necessary to reach the recommended duration.

Finally, remember to warm-up before stretching (this increases blood flow to muscles, ligaments, and tendons and makes them more pliable). Engage in a gentle, repetitive activity such as fast walking, running, skipping rope, stationary biking, or something similar until there is a light sweat.

Always observe proper technique to get maximum benefit and avoid injury. Many athletes become frustrated with flexibility programs because they do not see themselves making immediate gains. The problem is often poor technique. There are no shortcuts to achieving good flexibility; by trying to take shortcuts athletes will not improve their flexibility and may even injure themselves in the process. It is important to pay close attention to technique and to the duration of the stretch. Do not bounce or overstretch. Athletes often overstretch because they are eager to get the stretching phase over with. It is not necessary to be uncomfortable while stretching. A good exercise mat will increase comfort. Finally, there should be no pain felt during a stretch. If the athlete feels pain, he or she may be overstretching and should reduce the length of the stretch.

STRETCHING EXERCISES

The following exercises make up part of a safe and effective flexibility program that you can use for your prerun stretch routine.

INNER HIP: BUTTERFLY LEAN

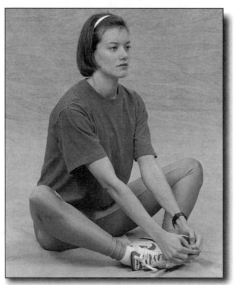

Sit with the soles of your feet together and lean forward, keeping your back straight.

TRUNK: SIDE STRETCH

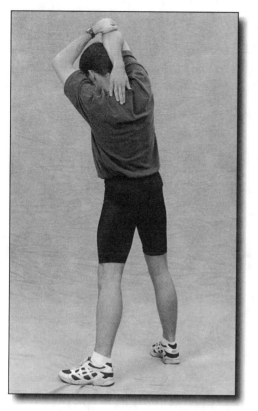

Stand with your right arm raised. Grasp your right elbow with your left hand behind your head and gently pull your right arm to your ear. Bend your trunk to the left until you feel stretch in your upper back and trunk. Hold for 60 seconds; then repeat on your other side.

BACK OF THE HIP: SITTING TOE TOUCH

Sit with your legs straight out in front of you. Keeping your back straight, lean forward from the hips, and with your arms extended, reach toward your toes.

QUADRICEPS: STANDING BALLET STRETCH

Stand on your left leg. With your left arm, balance yourself using a chair or wall. Bend your right leg back and pull your right ankle up toward your right buttock. With your right hand, pull up on your ankle so that your knee points down until you feel the action point. Hold for 60 seconds and then change sides.

FRONT OF THE HIP: LUNGE

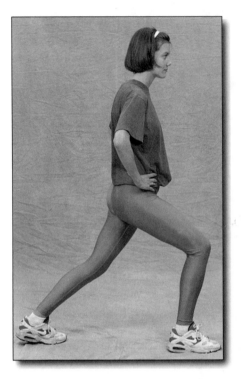

Begin with the feet together, hands on your hips, and eyes focused straight ahead. With your right foot take a big step forward. Your front foot should face straight ahead. Your back foot should also face forward, but the heel should be off the ground. Keep your shoulders back, your hips straight, and your eyes forward. Bend your forward knee, moving your pelvis forward toward the floor until you feel the action point. You should feel this stretch in the quadriceps of your back leg and in the front of that hip. Hold the stretch on each side for 60 seconds. Make this exercise more difficult by placing your forward foot on a chair or bench.

HAMSTRINGS: SEATED PIKED HAMSTRING STRETCH

Sit on the floor with your legs outstretched, ankles together, and toes pointed upward. Place your hands on the floor by the thighs. Look straight ahead and gently slide your hands forward. Keep your back and knees straight and try to bring your chest as close to your knees and thighs as possible. When you feel a stretch behind your knees and thighs, stop and hold this position for 60 seconds.

ANKLES: TOE CIRCLES

Sit with your knees fully straightened, your toes pointing up, and your ankles 12 inches apart. Relax your thigh and leg muscles. Begin by pointing your toes away from you. Rotate your feet away from each other in a circular motion. Make the largest circles you can. Perform 15 circles in one direction; then do 15 in the other direction. Repeat the exercise with your feet pointed back toward your knees.

OUTER HIP: STANDING LATERAL LEAN

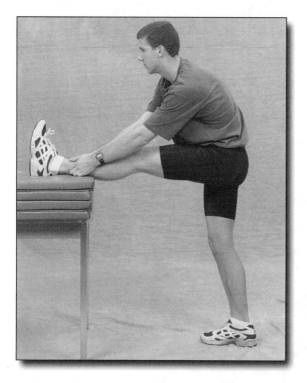

Place the foot of one leg on a table that is approximately the same height as your hips. Keeping both legs straight, lean toward the raised leg. Repeat with the other leg.

FRONT AND OUTSIDE OF THIGH: LYING QUADRICEPS AND ILIOTIBIAL BAND STRETCH

Lie on your left side with your left knee bent at 90 degrees and your right leg straight. Then bend your right leg and grasp that ankle with your

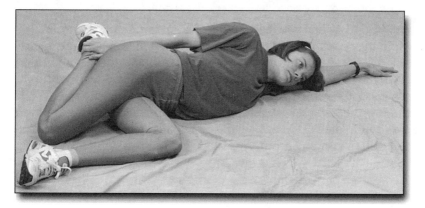

right hand. Gently pull your right heel toward your right buttocks. When you feel the stretch in your right quadriceps, lower your knee toward the floor in back of your left knee. Hold for 60 seconds. This will produce a stretch in the muscles around the hip (known as the tensor fascia lata and the iliotibial band) as well as in the quadriceps. Repeat on the other side.

CALVES AND ACHILLES TENDONS: WALL CALF STRETCH

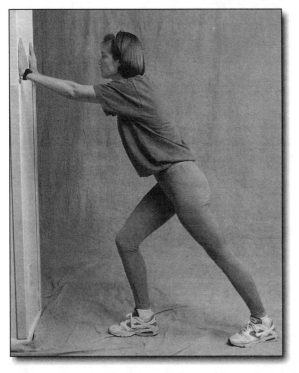

Stand an arm's length away from a wall or post you can lean on for balance, with your feet shoulder-width apart. Slowly slide your left foot directly back approximately two feet, keeping your left leg fully extended and your foot pointed slightly inward. The heels of both feet should stay flat on the floor. Look directly forward, and keep your hips and shoulders squared. Bend your right knee and slowly move your pelvis forward. When you feel a stretch in your left Achilles tendon, stop and hold the position for 60 seconds. Switch legs and repeat the exercise.

You can also perform this exercise by standing with feet shoulder-width apart and slightly turned in. Leaning against a wall with outstretched hands, allow your body to fall forward toward the wall. While keeping your back and knees straight, move your chest and hips toward the wall until you feel a stretch in the upper calf area. Hold this position for 60 seconds. As you become more flexible, you can stand farther from the wall.

The second part of this exercise emphasizes the Achilles tendon.

Stand an arm's length from a wall with the feet shoulder-width apart. Slide your right foot directly back about 18 inches. While keeping the heels of both feet flat on the ground, gently bend both knees until you feel a stretch in the calf and Achilles tendon of your back leg. Hold this position for 60 seconds and repeat for the left leg.

HAMSTRINGS AND GROIN: WALL SPLIT

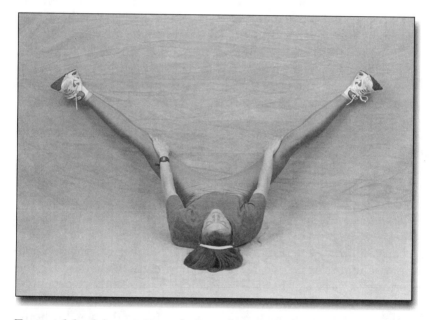

To stretch both hamstrings, the lower back, and hip adductors, begin by lying beside a wall. Bend the knees; then swing around so your body is at a right angle to the wall. Raise both legs so that your buttocks are flat against the wall, your legs are pointing up, and your feet are resting against the wall (if the hamstrings are so tight that the buttocks cannot reach the wall, start one or two feet away from the wall). Straighten the knees to stretch the hamstring and calf muscles. Then, while keeping your knees straight, gently slide your legs apart and allow gravity to pull your feet toward the floor. Continue to let your feet slide down the wall until you feel a stretch on the inner thigh. Hold each position for 60 seconds.

Strength Training

Whether an athlete uses free weights (barbells or dumbbells) or machines to strength train, he or she should consider the key elements of frequency and intensity when developing a strength training program.

Frequency: Do three workouts per week with a day of rest between each workout. Muscles need time to recover from a strength training session. A day without strength training is needed because the muscle-protein synthesis that produces increases in size and strength occurs during rest, not during the actual exercise. Athletes should not subscribe to the notion that if a little bit is good, a lot must be better.

Intensity: Intensity is gauged by the size of the weight and the number of repetitions performed. A muscle develops strength by adapting to greater demands, both in daily activities and by artificial methods such as training with weights. The greater the intensity, the greater the increase in strength. This is known as the overload principle. However, using weights that are too heavy may impair strength development and cause injury. Proper intensity is critical to achieving strength gains without pain.

Individuals train at different levels of intensity. The general guideline is that the weight should be between 50 and 80 percent of the athlete's maximum lift (known as 1RM). Whenever the weight is increased, the number of repetitions should be decreased. If not, technique is likely to suffer because the athlete will be struggling toward the end of the set, thus increasing the risk of injuring muscles and joints. The athlete should increase the amount of weight gradually and only when he or she is ready. It is time to increase the weight when the athlete can comfortably perform the maximum number of sets and maximum repetitions. Athletes can increase the weight when they are able to perform three sets of 12 repetitions for two consecutive workouts.

Intensity also includes the speed at which exercises should be done. For runners, the 2-4 system is most effective: lifting the weight should take 2 seconds, and lowering it should take 4 seconds. This gives enough time for both exercising and rest periods. Between sets, the athlete should take between 15 and 60 seconds of rest.

Comparing Strength Training Equipment

There are three basic types of strength training equipment: *free weights* (such as barbells, dumbbells, ankle/wrist weights), *vari-*

(continued)

able resistance machines (such as Keiser, Nautilus, and Universal), and *accommodating resistance machines* (Cybex, Lido, Kin-Com, among others). The exercises in this chapter are demonstrated with free weights, though all three types of equipment are useful for increasing muscle size and strength so long as the basic strength training guidelines are observed (see the next page). With the variety of strength training equipment now available, it is worthwhile for athletes to know the advantages and disadvantages of all three kinds.

Free weights can strengthen multiple muscle groups using just one weight. They also strengthen both eccentric contractions (lengthening of the muscles during the lowering phase) and concentric contractions (shortening of the muscles during the lifting phase), which prepares the muscle for any type of sports action, not just for a specific strength training motion. In general, free weights also provide a versatile and inexpensive form of isotonic exercise. Also, they do not take up much space.

The main disadvantages of free weights are (1) that changing the resistance can be cumbersome and time consuming and (2) if the athlete becomes tired or does not know proper strength training technique, free weights can be dangerous (a spotter is usually recommended).

Variable resistance machines apply isotonic stress to a muscle through its entire range of motion. Both eccentric and concentric contractions are strengthened, and the machines are safe, quick, and easy to adjust.

However, the routines offered by these machines are often not sport-specific. Weight increases may be too large for beginners or too small for the very strong. These machines are expensive, and they often do not fit small people very well.

Accommodating resistance machines work using controlled speed and resistance. The isokinetic workouts can be individualized to take into consideration a person's strengths and weaknesses throughout the entire range of motion. In addition, specific muscles can be isolated. Since it is usually not possible

(continued)

to overexert the muscles using these machines, they are especially useful for rehabilitation.

Again, the routines available are not sport-specific. Eccentric contractions are not strengthened and muscle involvement may be isolated. These machines are extremely expensive.

STRENGTHENING EXERCISES

When performing strength training exercises, the athlete should

- always use proper technique,
- always perform an exercise through the full range of motion, and
- always have total control over the weight, moving it in a smooth, fluid motion.

BENT-KNEE CRUNCHES: ABDOMINALS

Lie on the floor with your knees bent, holding a weight plate behind your head or on your upper chest. Slowly lift your head and shoulders off the floor while pressing the lower back into the floor. Pause; then lower your head and shoulders to the floor.

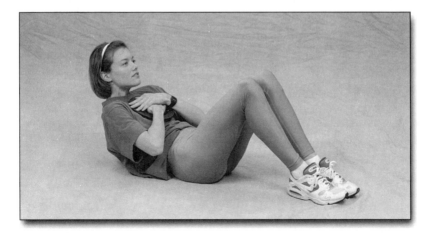

Barbell Squat: Quadriceps, Hamstrings, Buttocks, Lower Back

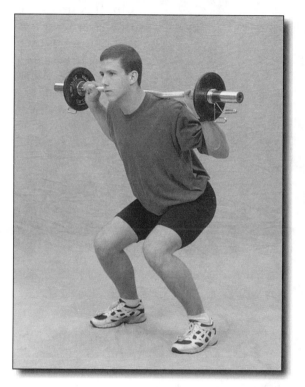

Stand with the feet shoulder-width apart and the barbell placed across your shoulders. Keeping your back straight and looking straight ahead, slowly lower your hips until your thighs are almost parallel with the floor. Pause; then return to the standing position.

Barbell Heel Raise: Calves

Stand with your toes on a raised surface, your feet shoulder-width apart, and the barbell across your shoulders. Keeping your back straight and looking straight ahead, slowly raise your heels as high as possible, pause, and then return to the starting position.

TUBED LEG SWING: HIPS

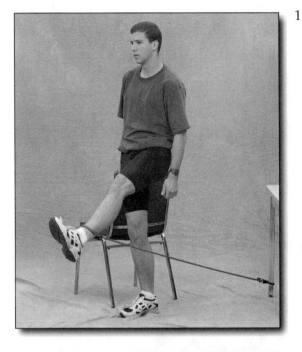

1. To strengthen the hip flexors, loop tubing around one ankle, and attach the other end to a fixed object. With your back to the anchor, support yourself with one hand and raise your leg until your thigh is almost parallel with the floor. Keep your knee straight, back erect, and do not bend forward or backward.

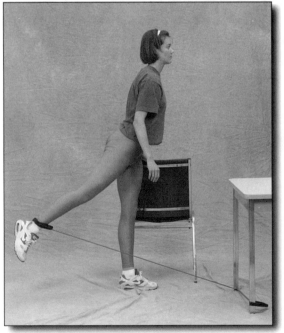

2. To strengthen the hip extensors, do the same exercise as above, this time facing the anchor.

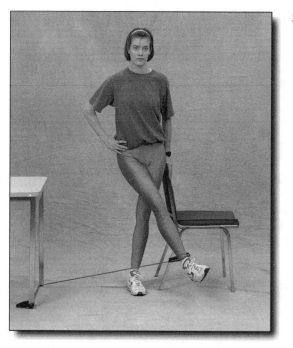

3. To strengthen the hip adductors, do the same exercise as above, this time standing sideways to the anchor with the tubing attached to the closer leg. Swing the leg across the body.

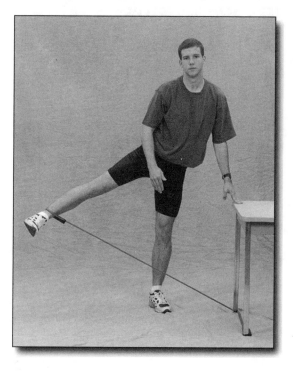

4. To strengthen the hip abductors, do the same exercise as above, this time with the tubing attached to the leg farther from the anchor, and raise your leg away from your body.

TOE RAISE: SHINS

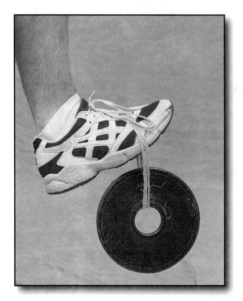

Sit on a raised surface so your knee is at a right angle. Attach a weight plate to your foot with a rope. Slowly raise your foot toward your shins as far as possible, pause, and then return to the starting position.

TUBED ANKLE EVERTERS AND INVERTERS*

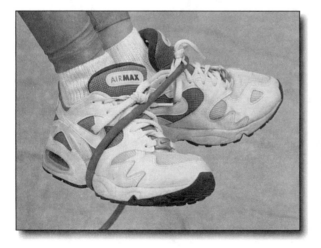

Sit with your legs together and wrap the tubing around your feet. Pull the fronts of your feet apart, pushing against the tubing; then pull your heels apart. Repeat 10 times. Next, flex one foot at a time, up and down, 10 times each. Cross

---

*For exercises to strengthen the hips and the ankle inverters and everters, athletes will need rubber tubes. Athletes can use either surgical tubing (available at surgical supply stores) or special conditioning tubing (Lifeline Gym Cord and Sports Cord are two reputable brands).

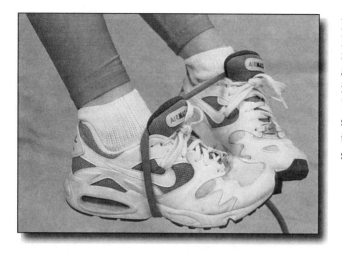

your ankles and push the top foot outward and bottom foot inward. Repeat 10 times; then switch feet. Do two to three sets.

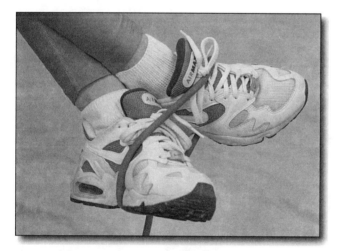

A CONDITIONING PROGRAM FOR THE BACK

The lower-back conditioning program described here goes beyond the traditional sit-ups for abdominal strength and modified hurdler's stretch for the hamstrings. It includes exercises for all five major anatomical areas. The runner should perform all the exercises since ignoring any anatomical area may lead to imbalances.

The following exercises for the five anatomical areas are presented in three degrees of difficulty—beginner, intermediate, and advanced. Make selections from each group, depending on fitness level, and do the exercises at least once a day.

LOWER BACK FLEXIBILITY

Beginner – KNEE TO CHEST

Lying on your back, bring one or both knees to your chest, grasp the leg under the thigh(s), and raise and lower your head slowly. Do the stretch slowly and hold it for 10 to 60 seconds.

Intermediate – "MAD CAT"

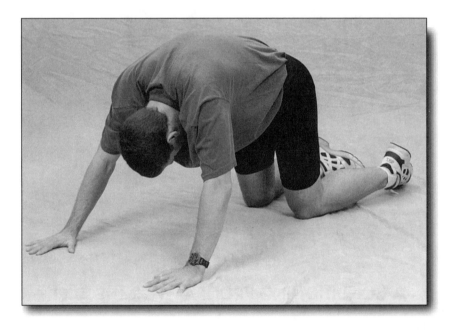

Kneeling on all fours, look up with your back dipped; then move so you are looking down and your back is humped. Do the stretch slowly and hold it for 10 to 60 seconds.

Advanced – CROSSED LEG FLEXION

Sit with your knees flexed and your ankles crossed. Slowly bend forward so your head approaches the floor. Do the stretch slowly and hold it for 10 to 60 seconds.

HAMSTRING FLEXIBILITY

Beginner –MODIFIED HURDLER'S STRETCH

Sit with one leg straight out and the other flexed. Move the flexed knee to the side and bend forward. Change sides. Do the stretch slowly and hold it for 10 to 60 seconds.

Intermediate –SUPINE POSITION

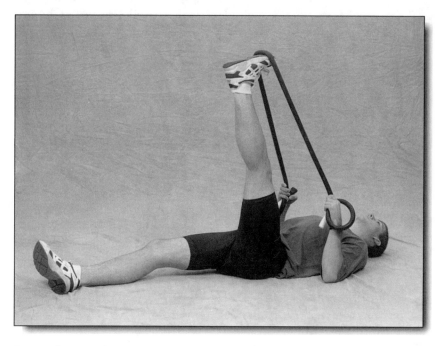

Lying down, place a jump rope around your foot or ankle; then raise your leg straight into the air. Contract the hamstring muscle against the tension of the rope, relax, and then pull the leg straighter. Change sides. Do the stretch slowly and hold it for 10 to 60 seconds.

Advanced –STANDING STRETCH

Stand with one leg on a support so the hip is flexed at 90 degrees. Keeping your back straight and your shoulders back, lean forward. Do the stretch slowly and hold it for 10 to 60 seconds.

HIP FLEXOR FLEXIBILITY

Beginner –HIP EXTENSION

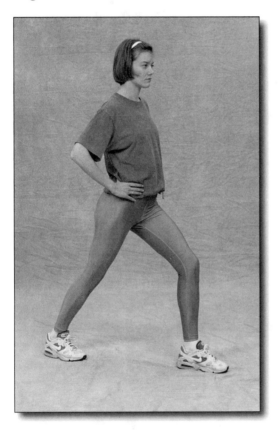

Stand with your pelvis in a neutral position. Extend your leg backward from the hip. Do the stretch slowly and hold it for 10 to 60 seconds. Change sides.

Advanced –LYING STRETCH

Lie on a bench with your knees over the edge and your back flat. Pull one leg to the chest to stretch the opposite hip. Do the stretch slowly and hold for 10 to 60 seconds. Change sides.

ABDOMINAL STRENGTH AND ENDURANCE

Beginner –PELVIC TILT

Lying down or standing with the back against a wall, press pelvis to the floor or wall. Repeat in a controlled manner 5 to 25 times.

Intermediate –PARTIAL CURL (CRUNCH)

Lying down with your knees flexed, curl up while sliding your hands by your sides a distance of three to four inches. Repeat in a controlled manner 5 to 25 times.

Advanced –OBLIQUE CURL

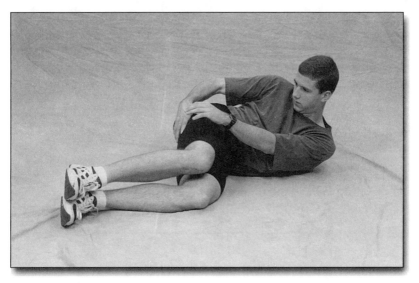

Lying on your side, twist your torso and curl up, reaching for your top leg with your opposite arm. Repeat in a controlled manner 5 to 25 times.

BACK EXTENSOR STRENGTH AND ENDURANCE

Beginner –HYPEREXTENSION I

Lie on your stomach with your hands by your sides. Keeping your neck and chin in a neutral position, raise your shoulders off the ground. Repeat in a controlled manner 5 to 25 times.

Intermediate –HYPEREXTENSION II

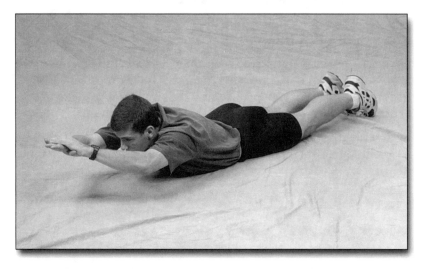

Lie on your stomach with your arms and hands extended forward. Keeping your neck and head in a neutral position, raise your shoulders off the floor. Repeat in a controlled manner 5 to 25 times.

Advanced –HYPEREXTENSION III

Lie on your stomach on a bench, positioning yourself so your body is supported from the pelvis down. Bend your waist to 90 degrees so your head is moving toward the floor; then bend it upward to several inches above horizontal. Repeat in a controlled manner 5 to 25 times.

Bursitis

Bursae are small pouches of fluid found in parts of the body where friction and stress occur. They are found

- between a bone and a tendon (e.g., the subacromial bursa between the rotator cuff tendon and acromioclavicular joint of the shoulder),
- between two tendons (e.g., the octocalcaneal bursa between the calcaneous and Achilles tendons in the heel), or
- between a bone and the skin (e.g., olecranon bursa between the point of the elbow and the skin).

(continued)

An overuse bursa injury, known as bursitis, occurs when irritation of the bursa causes fluid to flow into the sac and become inflamed. In a bursa that lies between two tendons or between a tendon and a bone, irritation is usually caused by repetitive movement of the tendon over the bursa.

Preventing bursitis

Prevent bursitis from developing in the first place by following these guidelines:

- Wear appropriate protective equipment to prevent repetitive microtrauma to the bursa in sports where such recurrent stress is likely.
- Make sure equipment is not responsible for causing bursitis (calcaneal bursitis behind the heel, for instance, is often caused by rubbing of the back of improperly fitting shoes against the heel).
- Embark on a strength and flexibility program to prevent irritation of the bursae by weak, tight tendons.
- Do a proper warm-up and cool-down to prevent tightness in the tendons that can cause irritation of the bursae.

If bursitis develops, prevent it from deteriorating into a chronic condition by following these guidelines:

- Protect it from further impact.
- Use the RICE prescription.
- Take acetaminophen or ibuprofen as label-directed.
- Seek medical care if the bursitis doesn't go away in a week.

If a chronic condition develops, prevent it from becoming permanently dysfunctional by seeking medical attention—probably anti-inflammatory medication, steroid injection into the bursa, and possibly surgical removal of the bursa.

Guard Against Nutritional Abuse

Female runners, especially those who exercise primarily for weight control, must be wary of disordered eating habits and their effect on menstrual regularity. For more information on avoiding complications caused by menstrual irregularity, see chapter 10.

Addressing Extrinsic Risk Factors

Because the athlete can more easily control them, extrinsic risk factors are generally easier to address than intrinsic risk factors. The following sections offer effective ways of dealing with risk factors associated with running.

Structure Your Workout Properly

Without properly preparing for the physical demands of running, runners are at a greatly increased risk of developing an overuse injury.

Every running session should include 5 minutes of limbering up, 5 to 10 minutes of stretching, 10 minutes of warm-up, and after the run, 10 minutes of cool-down and cool-down stretching.

Limbering Up (5 minutes)

Muscles must be warmed up before they can be safely and effectively stretched. Raising the body temperature makes the muscles more lubricated and elastic, increases secretions in the joints, and thus reduces friction. Ideal limbering-up exercises include light jogging, stationary bike riding, brisk walking, rope skipping, and using a rowing machine or stairclimber.

It is unnecessary to become tired during the limbering-up phase. The limbering-up stage is complete when the runner breaks a sweat.

Stretching (5 to 10 minutes)

The runner should do 5 to 10 minutes of stretching exercises after the limbering-up period.

Refer to pages 32-37 for a series of stretches that should be done before exercising. Follow the guidelines carefully. Do not overstretch, and remember to hold each stretch for between 30 and 60 seconds. Do each stretch one, two, or three times, depending on preexisting levels of flexibility, area-specific tightness, and previous injuries.

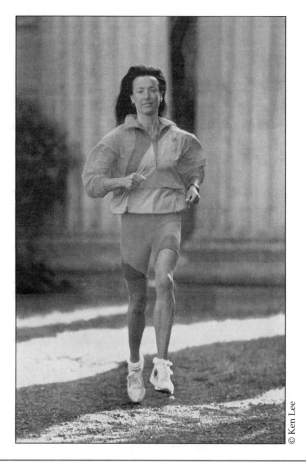

© Ken Lee

Raising body temperature *before* stretching is the safest and most effective way to enhance flexibility.

Warming Up Prior to Vigorous Activity

The warm-up should ideally last 10 minutes. An effective warm-up for a runner is to start with a walk-jog and then slowly increase speed to a run. When warming up for running, the heart rate should be 50 percent of maximum heart rate.

Cooling Down (5 minutes) and Cool-Down Stretches (5 minutes)

Ending a long run suddenly can cause light-headedness or even fainting. A 5-minute cooling down period avoids sudden changes that can cause such problems.

The purpose of the cool-down is to let the heart rate return to normal. Toward the end of the run runners should gradually slow down to a walk. If engaged in competition, continue to walk briskly after reaching the finishing line.

Stretching is also part of the cool-down period. Stretching for 5 minutes after a run prevents muscles from tightening too quickly. It lessens muscle discomfort and can help maintain general flexibility.

Although most athletes recognize the need for a properly structured workout session, many neglect this crucial aspect of preventive sports care. As a result, many become injured. In this fast-paced world, it is difficult enough to find time to exercise, let alone find the time for pre- and postexercise workout regimens. But it is crucial for a person participating in vigorous exercise to structure a workout properly. From an injury standpoint, no exercise session at all is better than a poorly organized one.

Joint/Cartilage Injuries

Joints are where the ends of two bones meet. Joints act as levers that, when operated by muscle movements, set our bodies in motion. Without joints, it would be impossible to perform even the simplest of movements.

Ninety percent of the joints are freely movable joints, or synovial joints, where the ball at the end of one bone meets the socket of another. Synovial joints are the biggest joints, and the ones most often injured in sports.

The ball-and-socket structure of the joints provides them with the mechanism to move. But the joints can only move smoothly because of the presence of cartilage.

Articular cartilage is a thin coating at the ends of the two bones that meet to form the joint. It is extremely tough, yet well lubricated. The presence of articular cartilage lets our joints move smoothly. When injured, damaged articular cartilage interferes with joint movement. The gradual erosion of articular cartilage is responsible for the condition known as degenerative arthritis.

A meniscus is a flat, crescent-shaped piece of cartilage present in about 10 percent of the joints. Menisci stabilize the joint, absorb shock, and disperse lubrication known as synovial fluid. Blood supply to the meniscus is very poor, and it has no nerves or lympathic channels. That makes it virtually impossible for

(continued)

an injured meniscus to heal itself. Considering the amount of stress the knee undergoes during sports, and the inability of the meniscus to heal itself, it is not surprising that a torn knee meniscus is one of the most common athletic injuries.

The joint's hard tissues (the bone, cartilage, and articular cartilage) can become injured in sports in two ways—through massive trauma and through repetitive, low-intensity trauma damages to these tissues. Because running is not a sport that causes acute injuries, only overuse injuries will be covered in this section.

Overuse joint/cartilage injuries are common among runners. They are caused by the wear and tear running exerts on joints in the lower extremities. Joint/cartilage damage not only puts runners out of sports, but also leads to arthritis in later life. For this reason, prompt diagnosis and proper treatment of these kinds of injuries is very important. Because cartilage has no blood supply, it cannot heal itself. For that reason, surgery is often necessary for joint/cartilage injuries.

Injury types

The two most common overuse joint/cartilage injuries are osteochondritis dissecans (loose bodies in the joint) and meniscus tears (damage to the meniscus cartilage between the joints).

Preventing osteochondritis dissecans

Prevent osteochondritis dissecans from happening in the first place by following these guidelines:

- Observe a progressive training regimen to minimize sudden increases in stress to the joint surface.
- Develop flexibility in the joint and surrounding ligaments and tendons to minimize grinding together of the joint surfaces.

If this condition develops, prevent lesions of the joint surface from breaking off and forming loose bodies in the joint by following these guidelines:

- Cease running as soon as symptoms are felt.
- Use the RICE prescription.
- Take acetaminophen or ibuprofen as label-directed.

(continued)

- Seek expert orthopedic care.
- Carefully follow the rehabilitation program.
- Do not return to running until the doctor and the physical therapist provide clearance.

If loose bodies enter the joint (full-blown osteochondritis dissecans), prevent permanent joint dysfunction by following these guidelines:

- Seek expert orthopedic care for probable surgical intervention.
- Carefully follow the postsurgery rehabilitation program.

Preventing meniscus tears

Prevent meniscus tears from happening in the first place by following these guidelines:

- Observe a progressive training regimen to minimize sudden increases in stress to the joints.
- Develop strength and flexibility in the joint and surrounding ligaments and tendons to reduce compression and twisting forces that damage the meniscus.

When the early symptoms of this condition are felt, prevent minor tears from deteriorating into complete ruptures of the meniscus by following these guidelines:

- Cease running.
- Use the RICE prescription.
- Take acetaminophen or ibuprofen as label-directed.
- Seek expert orthopedic care.
- Carefully follow the rehabilitation program.
- Do not return to running until the doctor and the physical therapist provide clearance.

If the meniscus renders the joint completely useless, prevent permanent joint dysfunction by following these guidelines:

- Seek expert orthopedic care for probable surgical intervention.
- Carefully follow the postsurgery rehabilitation program.
- Do not return to running until the doctor and the physical therapist provide clearance.

Avoid Training Errors

Beginning runners are at especially high risk of developing overuse injuries because their bodies are relatively deconditioned. While increases in heart and lung endurance can be achieved quickly through running, increases in bone and soft tissue strength take place more slowly, putting the beginning runner at risk of injuries to these structures. Tendinitis conditions and stress fractures of the bones are thus seen often in beginning runners.

Overuse injuries do not occur only in novice runners or recreational runners who run regularly. A nationally ranked runner who had been training more than 90 miles a week dropped below 70 miles a week during a three-week period of university finals. He then resumed his 90-miles-per-week pace. As a result of this sudden increase in mileage, he sustained a stress fracture of his shin bone.

It is usually safe to increase either the frequency, duration, or intensity of the exercise regimen by 10 percent without making adjustments (the 10 percent rule). But when dramatically increasing the volume of one of the three elements of the exercise regimen, it is necessary to make temporary adjustments in one or both of the other elements.

Increase in exercise duration = reduce frequency and/or intensity.

Increase in exercise frequency = reduce duration and/or intensity.

Increase in exercise intensity = reduce duration and/or frequency.

By how much, though, should athletes cut back? When athletes intensify one element of their exercise regimen, they should cut back on one of the other two elements by 20 percent, and then increase it by 5 percent each week until it reaches its previous level. For instance, a jogger runs five miles in an hour every other day on grass. If he switches from grass to concrete (a change in intensity), he should reduce how long he runs.

The Sun's Harmful Rays

Sunburn, known in medical terminology as actinic dermatitis, is the destruction of skin cells caused by the sun's ultraviolet radiation. Most of us have suffered through sunburn sometime during childhood; for runners—and others who enjoy outdoor activities—low-intensity exposure can be a long-term threat.

(continued)

The symptoms of a sunburn usually show up two to three hours after exposure. Sunburns are classified according to their severity—first, second, or third degree—and the symptoms vary accordingly. With a first-degree sunburn, the skin turns pink to bright red. Sufferers of a second-degree burn will develop blisters. In third-degree sunburns, the skin may turn black or white, and there may be little pain. Fortunately, second-degree sunburns are rare, and third-degree sunburns are even rarer.

Aspirin is an extremely effective means of treating mild to moderate sunburn. Not only does the aspirin provide pain relief, it also blocks a biochemical reaction that causes the skin to redden, and shuts down the sun's damage to the skin. As soon as the burn is felt (it does not work the day after), take two aspirin and take two more every two to three hours to a maximum of eight. Children with sunburn can be given pediatric aspirin.

Aloe vera cream sold in drugstores provides effective, natural relief from sunburn. Do not use the anesthetic sprays available in drugstores. They provide temporary pain relief but dry out the skin and delay recovery.

Seek medical attention from a dermatologist when the skin is bright red, tender, and covered with blisters that weep and ooze. This is a sign of a second-degree burn. The doctor may remove the fluid from the blisters and prescribe an oral steroid cream such as prednisone to be used for several days.

Sunburn is one of the most easily prevented skin problems. Any athlete who participates in outdoor sports should use a sunscreen. All sunscreens now come with sun protection factor (SPF) ratings, from 2 to 45. These ratings let consumers know how long they can stay in the sun before burning when using the sunscreen versus using no protection. For example, someone who would normally start to turn pink in 20 minutes can use an SPF 10 sunscreen and withstand up to 200 minutes of sun exposure without getting burned.

An SPF-15 provides enough protection for most people. But for people who have fair skin, blue eyes, freckles, and either blond or red hair, a higher-numbered SPF may be appropriate.

It is essential that the sunscreen be waterproof so it does not wash off in contact with perspiration, swimming water, or water used to cool off during a workout. Apply the sunscreen to

(continued)

dry skin after showering the morning before the athletic activity and reapply it just before exercising.

A sunburn can potentially cause a malfunctioning of the organs below the skin that can result in an infection of hair follicles or sweat glands. Incontrovertible evidence now shows that long-term, low-intensity exposure to strong sun can cause skin cancers that may be disfiguring or even fatal.

Any pain or joint stiffness should be a warning that the runner is increasing the other elements too quickly, and he or she should make further cutbacks.

Most runners engaged in endurance sports are primarily interested in improving their health. But many others are competitive athletes who wish to improve performance in endurance sports for personal satisfaction or competition.

The principle of improving endurance is based on overload—when the training load exceeds the accustomed work load. However, this works only up to a point. Competitive distance runners eventually reach a point when no further increase in endurance takes place. In fact, when runners continue pushing themselves to improve their performance beyond this maximal performance level, their performance may worsen. More significantly, injuries may occur. Overuse injuries are an inevitable outgrowth of overtraining to increase performance.

Competitive runners who wish to improve their performance should follow these guidelines:

- Do not increase training frequency, duration, or intensity by more than 10 percent per week.
- If performance stabilizes or worsens, or any of the symptoms of staleness becomes apparent, cut back on the training routine. Symptoms of injury such as swelling, increasing discomfort, or persistent pain are a signal to stop training and consult a sports doctor.
- Alternate hard workouts with easy ones. Give the body a rest between especially hard training days.
- To improve performance, do not just look to increasing distance or time; consider improvements in areas such as nutrition and technique.
- Do not begin as a competitive runner by training for the hardest race. For instance, those who want to be competitive runners should start by training for 3K races, not marathons.
- Use common sense to tell how much is too much.

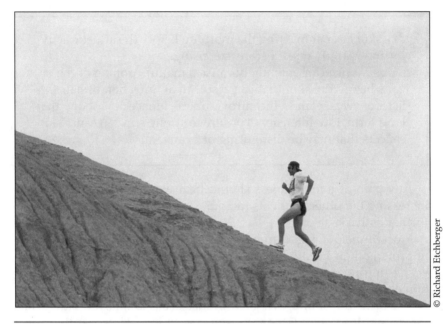

Performance may actually worsen if runners try to push the overload principle too far.

Bone Injuries

The human body has 206 bones that provide its skeletal framework. Overuse bone injuries are called stress fractures—tiny cracks in the bone surface caused by repetitive impact such as the pounding of the feet against the pavement. A series of identical events—rhythmic, repetitive, subthreshold trauma—causes stress fractures. Stress fractures are seen frequently in the feet and lower legs of runners.

Preventing stress fractures

Prevent stress fractures from happening in the first place by following these guidelines:

- Have a presports physical to determine whether there are any risk factors that might increase the risk of stress fractures.
- Observe a progressive training regimen that doesn't overstress the bones through sudden increases in the frequency, intensity, or duration.

(continued)

- Embark on a conditioning program to develop strength and flexibility in the bones and surrounding structures.
- Use the right equipment, especially footwear, and observe correct technique, especially in jogging and strength training.

If the symptoms of a stress fracture develop, prevent the injury from becoming a chronic condition by following these guidelines:

- Cease running.
- Use the RICE prescription.
- Take acetaminophen or ibuprofen as label-directed.
- Do not return to running until there is absolutely no pain in the area.
- Seek medical attention if the stress fracture symptoms are still present in two weeks.

If the stress fracture has become a chronic condition, prevent it from making the area permanently dysfunctional by seeking expert orthopedic care.

Wear Appropriate Footwear

Today's running shoes are far superior to those of just a decade ago. There is a strong emphasis on efficient biomechanical design and injury prevention measures. Choosing the right running shoe can still cause confusion, especially for those runners who have atypical foot types.

The following are the American Running and Fitness Association's guidelines for choosing the right running shoe. First, runners should know the five basic running shoe components: last, upper, outsole, midsole, and heel counter.

Last: The three-dimensional model on which the shoe is based.

Upper: The main portion of the shoe that surrounds the foot. Uppers used to be made of leather, but today they are made of synthetic fabrics that are lighter, washable, breathable, and require little or no break-in.

Outsole: The treaded layer glued to the bottom of the midsole. It resists wear, provides traction, and absorbs shock.

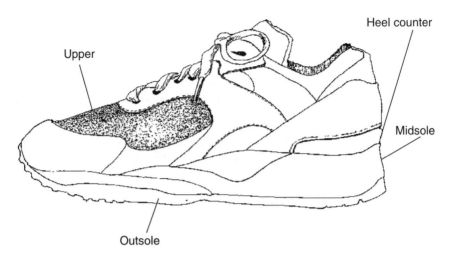

Upper

Heel counter

Midsole

Outsole

Midsole: Located between the outsole and the upper. It controls excessive foot motion and provides cushioning and shock absorption.

Heel counter: The inflexible material surrounding the heel. It must be rigid and durable to support and stabilize the heel.

First, the runner should find out if he or she is a pronator or a supinator. The runner can perform a self-test to determine foot type by bending halfway at the knees and noting the movement of the kneecaps. If the kneecaps move toward the inside of the feet, the runner is probably a pronator. If the kneecaps point slightly outward, he or she probably has supinating feet.

A pronator's foot rolls inward too much when running. Pronators tend to have flexible feet, which can cause injuries such as kneecap pain, iliotibial band syndrome, and tendinitis.

A pronator should get a shoe that is board-lasted. The last and the upper are attached using three techniques, one of which is board-lasting. In board-lasting, the upper materials are pulled over the last and the ends are glued or stitched to the bottom. A board-lasted shoe is very supportive, which is ideal for the pronator.

A supinator's foot rolls outward when running. Supinators tend to have rigid feet and cannot absorb shock as well as pronators, so the supinator is more susceptible to ankle sprains, stress fractures, and pain on the outside of the shin and knee. Excessive supination does not occur often.

A supinator should look for a slip-lasted shoe or a combination-lasted shoe. In slip-lasting, the upper material circles the last, with the edges stitched together on the bottom. Slip-lasting is light and flexible. Combination-lasting is done using two methods, with the board process in the heel and slip process in the forefoot. This construction provides stiffness, with flexibility in the toe area.

If a person bends halfway at the knees and the kneecaps point in the same direction as the feet, then he or she is neither a pronator nor a

Exercise Tips for Elders

Although people of all ages begin and maintain a running program in almost the same way, here are some tips for older runners from the American Running and Fitness Association.

- Have a complete physical examination (including a stress test) before starting. The exam should include a risk factor analysis to help determine whether you are susceptible to developing cardiovascular disease.
- Never skip the warm-up or cool-down. These activities help prevent injuries.
- Become familiar with your target heart rate—the rate at which your heart should beat while you exercise. If your doctor has not told you what your target heart rate is, you can figure it out yourself. Subtract your age from 220 and take 60 to 75 percent of that figure by multiplying by .60 and .75. Example for a 70-year-old: $220 - 70 = 150$, $150 \times .60 = 90$ beats per minute, $150 \times .75 = 112$ beats per minute. Thus, a 70-year-old's target heart rate is between 90 and 112 beats per minute.

While exercising, take your pulse (either at your wrist, or next to or on one side of your Adam's apple) for 15 seconds and multiply by four. That is your pulse, or heart rate, for one minute. Are you exercising at your target heart rate? Your pulse should not go beyond your target heart rate range.

You can also make sure you are not overexerting yourself by using the talk test, according to Charles Schulman, MD, assistant clinical professor of medicine at Harvard Medical School in Boston, and editorial board member for the American Running and Fitness Association. If you can talk comfortably while running, you are probably exercising at the appropriate pace.

- Start your running program *slowly*. If you become fatigued and feel you should stop, then stop for the day. Remember that you will not improve as fast as a younger person, so do not become discouraged. You will reach your goal— it just might take a few months instead of a few weeks. Do not overexert yourself.

(continued)

- Certain exercises are less stressful than others. Walking, for instance, may be a better alternative to running if you have not exercised in years. It burns about the same number of calories if the same distance is covered and gives you a good workout—especially if you stay within your target heart rate range.
- For all-around fitness, an aerobic exercise (one that works your lungs and cardiovascular system for at least 20 to 30 consecutive minutes) such as running is best, but find other healthful, enjoyable activities to complement your aerobic program. These could include gardening, horseshoe throwing, bowling, golf, tennis, croquet, hiking, or camping. Use these activities if you cannot exercise aerobically because of a medical disability. You might also want to try weight training with light weights or circuit weight training to help keep your bones strong. Talk with someone familiar with weights to help you.
- Remember that you must allow your body to recover from any type of exercise. After a workout, older people and formerly sedentary people of any age should allow their muscles to recover. One easy way to be sure you are rested is to exercise every other day. If you become injured or feel extra sore, take a break from your program and allow yourself to heal completely. Gentle walking, though, may be done on a daily basis.
- Try running with a partner or group of people who will help you get and stay motivated. You could, for example, become involved in a local mall-walking program, or a running or walking program sponsored by your local hospital or senior center.

supinator, and will not have to worry about buying a shoe with special features.

Whether someone is a pronator or a supinator, the following are the features all runners should look for in a running shoe:

- The shape of the last determines whether the runner has enough room for the longest toe to push forward naturally during each step. To determine which shape of last he or she needs—straight, semicurved, or curved—the runner must determine the shape of his or her foot. To evaluate foot shape, the runner should stand on a piece of paper and trace the outline of each foot. Superimpose the drawings on the soles of the shoes to see if the size and curvature are a good match.

• Make sure the shoe has a padded tongue to cushion against lace pressure and a padded ankle collar to cushion the ankle and help prevent Achilles tendinitis.

• For those who run on asphalt or cement, a ripple sole is recommended.

• For those who run on dirt or grass, stud or waffle outsoles are recommended because they improve traction and stability.

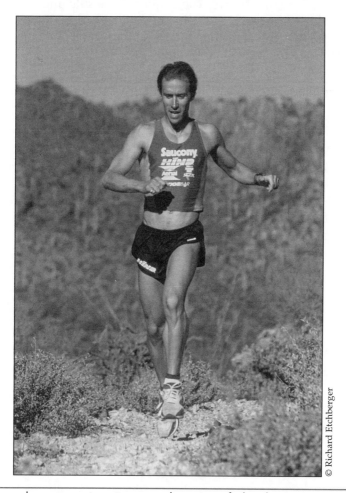

© Richard Etchberger

Where you choose to run is an important determiner of what shoe you wear.

- The runner should know what kind of midsole cushioning he or she is buying to predict how long the shoes will last. EVA (ethylene vinyl acetate) is a light foam with good cushioning, but it breaks down fairly quickly. Compression-molded EVA is harder and more durable than EVA. Many shoes are now cushioned with gel, air bags, silicone, and foam that are contained in a midsole of EVA or polyurethane (PU). This cushioning lasts longer than those produced by previous methods.

- The shoe should have a heel lift of about one-half to one inch. This enhances the shoe's ability to absorb shock and it reduces strains.

- Quality is an important factor. Before purchase, place the shoes on a flat surface at eye level. The midline of the heel counter should be perpendicular to the surface. The quality of the stitching, eyelets, and laces should also be checked. The buyer should check that the sole layers are evenly and completely glued to each other and to the upper. Check inside the shoe for lumps and bumps.

- The sole should flex easily where the foot flexes. Removable insoles are preferable so that they can be modified or replaced with orthotics.

For one dollar, the American Running and Fitness Association will send applicants a printout of running shoes that match individual needs. Call ARFA at 800-776-ARFA to get an order form.

Socks also count as footwear. They act as shock absorbers and protect the feet from rubbing against shoes. Socks should be thick to maximize impact absorption, free of holes to protect against blisters, and regularly laundered to avoid skin conditions. During the last 10 years a variety of heavyweight socks have helped reduce the incidence of impact- and friction-related injuries such as stress fractures, plantar fasciitis, and blisters.

Diagnosis and Management of Running Injuries

By following the preventive measures in the preceding chapter, many runners can avoid becoming injured. Yet it is inevitable that some runners will develop medical conditions related to their participation in running. Unfortunately, instead of addressing the problem early, there is a tendency among runners to dismiss the early symptoms of an overuse injury as just part of the normal aches and pains of running.

This is understandable. The symptoms of overuse injuries are slow to develop and often difficult to pinpoint. Initially, the runner may experience symptoms only after running. Gradually the runner may feel symptoms during and after a run, but they may not be severe enough to interfere with running performance. In the final stages, the runner will feel disabling pain both during and after running, and during daily activities.

What You Can Do to Manage Your Injury

Runners can treat their injuries so long as they are sure of the diagnosis. If runners are ever in doubt about the type of injury they may have, or if self-care measures fail to improve the condition within a reasonable amount of time (two to four weeks), they should see a sports doctor.

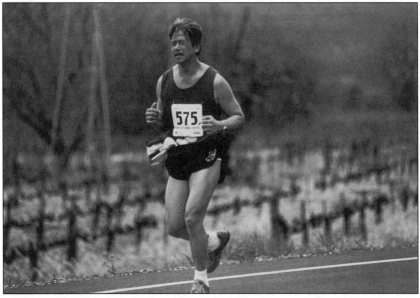

Symptoms of overuse injuries develop slowly and often only interfere with running performance in the final stages of injury.

Classifying Overuse Injuries

Below are the general guidelines for classifying overuse injuries according to severity, along with the appropriate response for each level of injury severity. The individual components of self-treatment and rehabilitation will be covered in subsequent sections.

Mild Injury

- Performance not affected
- Pain only after running
- Area not tender to touch
- No swelling or minimal swelling
- No discoloration

What You Should Do:

- Suspend running schedule, but continue strength and flexibility training that does not affect the injured area. Participate in alternative cardiovascular conditioning like cycling, swimming, or water running that will not compromise healing.

- Administer RICE (see pages 71-74) and over-the-counter (OTC) medication for 24 to 48 hours.
- After 24 hours, or when initial symptoms have abated, begin a strength and flexibility program for the affected area.
- In one week, resume running, starting at 75 percent of preinjury regimen intensity, and gradually working back to full intensity.

Moderate Injury

- Performance mildly affected
- Pain before and after running
- Area mildly tender to the touch
- Mild swelling
- Some discoloration

What You Should Do:

- Suspend running schedule, but continue strength and flexibility training that does not affect the injured area. Participate in cardio-vascular conditioning like cycling, swimming, or water running that will not compromise healing.
- Administer RICE and OTC medication for 48 to 72 hours.
- After 24 to 48 hours, or when initial symptoms have abated, begin moderate-intensity strength and flexibility exercises for the affected area, gradually increasing the intensity.
- In 7 to 10 days, resume running, starting at 50 percent of preinjury regimen intensity, and gradually working back to full intensity.

Severe Injury

- Pain before, during, and after running
- Performance affected by pain
- Normal movement affected by pain
- Pain when pressure applied to area
- Swelling
- Discoloration

What You Should Do:

- Suspend running schedule, but continue strength and flexibility training that does not affect the injured area and participate in cardiovascular conditioning that will not compromise healing.
- Administer RICE and OTC medication for three to seven days.

- After 48 hours, or when initial symptoms have abated, begin gentle strength and flexibility exercises for the affected area, gradually increasing the intensity.
- Resume running, starting at 25 to 50 percent of preinjury regimen intensity, if the following rehabilitation progression can be performed:

  1. Walk, first with small steps and then progress to bigger steps; when this becomes easy, walk around objects or in a "lazy z."
  2. Jog slowly in a straight line; then jog in a "lazy z" pattern and progress to a "sharp z."
  3. Sprint 5 to 10 meters, starting and stopping slowly, then more quickly. Trial run with the injury protected or supported where appropriate.

- If symptoms do not improve within two weeks, consult a sports doctor.

Coping With Allergies

The fall allergy season, beginning in late August and continuing until the first frost, affects many runners. Most allergic disease—"hay fever"—in the fall is triggered by ragweed pollen, especially in the Midwest and East.

Common symptoms are sneezing, watery eyes, runny nose, fatigue, headache, wheezing, coughing, nasal congestion, and itching in the throat, mouth, and ears. Some allergy sufferers also experience irritability, appetite loss, loss of concentration, and depression.

These symptoms differ in severity, depending on the amount of pollen in the air and on the weather. Dry, windy, sunny weather promotes allergic reactions in allergy sufferers.

Before resorting to prescription drugs or considering desensitization, runners should try these measures to alleviate unpleasant allergy symptoms:

- Avoid running in the morning and evening, when pollen settles near the ground.
- Keep windows closed and air-conditioning on at home to reduce the pollen level in the house. It is accumulated expo-

(continued)

sure to allergens that finally leads to allergic reactions. If the runner can protect himself or herself from exposure to pollen for at least eight hours every night, he or she may prevent the pollens from reaching a symptomatic level.

- Avoid insect sprays, fresh paint, tobacco smoke, and other substances that when inhaled can further irritate already inflammed membranes. Alcohol can also make allergy symptoms worse by dilating blood vessels.
- Over-the-counter antihistamines and decongestants may be necessary if one cannot avoid excessive exposure to pollens. If so, these drugs should be taken regularly to prevent symptoms rather than taken to relieve ongoing symptoms.
- Drink plenty of water to relieve the dryness of the mucous membranes caused by antihistamines.
- Maintain a well-balanced diet and a balanced program of running, recreation, and rest to help the body become more resistant to allergens in the air.

Apply RICE

Rest, Ice, Compression, and Elevation are the most important components of self-treatment for all athletes. Known under the acronym RICE, they are especially important after acute injuries such as ligament sprains or muscle bruises or strains. For runners, whose ailments tend to develop slowly and over time, RICE therapy is not as essential. However, runners can help alleviate the pain, inflammation, and swelling associated with overuse injuries by following this course of self-treatment.

Rest and Relative Rest

Running should cease as soon as overuse injury symptoms are felt. Continuing to run will only cause the injury to worsen and will result in long layoffs. Depending on how far the runner has allowed the injury to deteriorate, complete immobilization may be necessary for 24 to 72 hours to properly ice, compress, and elevate the injury.

After the initial stage of immobilization, rest does not mean total inactivity. Complete immobilization will only worsen the runner's health status by encouraging muscle atrophy, joint stiffness, and a decline in cardiovascular endurance. Runners can continue to participate in exercise that does not affect their injury; swimming, for instance, is an excellent nonweightbearing exercise for injured runners. Participating in exercise that does not interfere with recovery is known as relative rest, and will be covered in the section on rehabilitation.

Ice

Cooling the injury decreases swelling, bleeding, pain, and inflammation. The most effective way to do this is to apply ice to the affected area. For maximum effect, ice should be applied to the injury as early as possible. Characteristic sensations experienced when using ice are cold, a burning sensation, then aching, and finally numbness.

The most common method of icing an injury is by covering the injured area with a wet towel and placing a plastic bag full of ice over it. Wrap a bandage over the ice bag to keep it in place while simultaneously applying compression. The towel must be wet because a dry towel will serve to insulate the skin from the cooling effect.

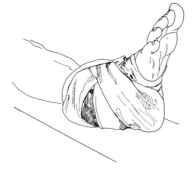

A less common but highly efficient method of icing an injury is ice massage. This is done by freezing water in a polystyrene coffee cup and then tearing off the upper edge of the cup. This leaves the base as an insulated grip, allowing the athlete to massage the injured area with slow, circular strokes. Ice massage combines two elements of RICE—icing and compression. Ice massage is especially effective for treating the symptoms of Achilles tendinitis.

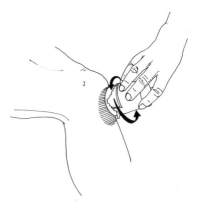

Although convenient, refrigerated commercial gel packs do not stay cold long enough and may leak dangerous chemicals if punctured.

In the past, icing was recommended for only 24 to 48 hours after symptoms were first felt. Evidence now suggests that intermittent icing may be beneficial for up to seven days. The first 72 hours are especially critical, and icing should be done as much as practically possible during this period. Ice the injury for 10 to 20 minutes at a time at intervals of 30 to 45 minutes.

Icing duration depends on the injured person's body type. In a thin person, significant muscle cooling occurs within 10 minutes, whereas fatter people may take 20 minutes to achieve comparable results.

An important caution is that one should *never apply ice to one area for more than 20 minutes.*

Compression

To reduce swelling, gentle but firm pressure should be applied to the injury. Compression can be performed while icing is being done and when it is not. During icing, perform simultaneous compression by doing ice massage with the coffee cup method. Alternatively, an elastic bandage can be wrapped over the ice pack and limb.

The following are important steps for applying an elastic bandage:

1. Start several inches below the injury (or away from the heart).
2. Wrap toward the heart in an overlapping spiral, starting with even and somewhat tight pressure, then gradually wrapping looser above the injury.
3. Periodically check the skin color, temperature, and sensation of the injured area to make sure the wrap isn't compressing any nerves or arteries.

Elevation

Keeping the injury elevated is necessary to combat gravitational forces that naturally pull blood and fluids toward it, where they collect and create swelling and inflammation.

Whenever possible, raise the injury above heart level. For example, an athlete with an ankle, knee, or thigh injury should lie on a couch or bed and use a pillow to keep the injury elevated. During the first 24 to 72 hours, elevate the injury whenever possible.

What You Should Not Do

During the first 24 to 48 hours, *do not*

- apply heat to the injured area (avoid hot showers and baths, liniments, etc.),
- massage the injury,
- exercise, or
- drink alcohol.

All of these can cause *increased* swelling and bleeding in the injured area.

Remember, RICE is a first aid treatment only. Depending on the nature and severity of the injury, it may be necessary to seek medical treatment.

Hyperthermia and Heat Exhaustion

During vigorous exercise, the amount of heat produced by the working muscles is 15 to 20 times what they produce at rest. As body temperature rises, the brain increases the amount of blood sent to the skin and stimulates sweating. If the cooling effect of sweating is inadequate—if the body produces heat at a faster rate than it can be dispersed—the person will overheat. Injury will occur when the body temperature goes higher than 104 degrees Farenheit.

During long runs the amount of body fluid lost through sweat can cause runners to become dehydrated. Severe dehydration causes a reduction in the athlete's capacity to sweat and therefore increases the risk of heat stroke, heat exhaustion, and muscle cramps. Children are especially susceptible to overheating and should be watched carefully during races.

The risk of heat injuries can be reduced by dressing properly for the weather. For example, light-colored clothing made of cotton is much better than dark-colored clothing made of synthetic fibers such as nylon. To reduce dehydration during long runs, drink plenty of fluids, mainly cool water.

In hot climates, athletes should avoid exercising outside when the sun is strongest. It is best to exercise in the early morning or late evening. Avoid strenuous workouts when the humidity is

(continued)

Warm-weather medical self-care for beginning runners[1]

Temperature is a critical factor. Significant heat injury may occur at temperatures above 65 degrees Farenheit. Above 80 degrees Farenheit, novice runners should reduce running pace by about one minute per mile. Wear only light athletic clothing (shorts, T-shirt, tank top, or topless). Body temperature will normally rise to 102 to 103 degrees Farenheit due to exercise heat production. Further increases may occur due to radiant sun exposure, dehydration, and decreased sweat rate.

Fluid replacement is essential to restore sweat losses. The average-size man (140 to 160 pounds) may lose 1.5 to 2.0 quarts of sweat per hour. Drink fluid during long runs. Stop to drink. Even then, you may replace only 50 percent of sweat loss.

Problems during a run may include muscle cramps, joint pains, blisters, and fatigue. Heat symptoms—headache, dizziness, disorientation, nausea, decrease in sweat rate, pale or cold skin—indicate danger of heat injury. Don't try to run through these symptoms. Stop and rest or walk.

At the completion of a run, you may become dizzy or faint on coming to a stop due to a fall in blood pressure. To prevent this, keep moving. If symptoms develop, lie down and raise your legs.

If you have medical problems such as asthma, diabetes, hypertension, or other cardiovascular problems, check with your physician. Wear a medic alert tag and ID.

Remember, running is fun but it can be stressful. Listen to your body. Walk when you are tired. There is always another day to run.

---

[1]Reprinted by permission, from P.G. Hanson, 1989, Heat injuries in runners: Treatment and prevention. In *Running injuries,* edited by D'Ambrosia and Drez (Thorofare, N.J.: Slack Incorporated), 196.

Over-the-Counter (OTC) Medications for Overuse Injuries

Over-the-counter pain relievers are an effective way to combat the effects of overuse injuries. However, the choices can be bewildering, so it is important to learn more about what is available.

The majority of over-the-counter pain relievers sold in the U.S. contain one of the following ingredients: acetaminophen, ibuprofen, or aspirin. At recommended doses, all three have about the same effect on reducing pain. For reducing pain *and* inflammation, only ibuprofen and aspirin are effective.

The following is a rundown of the common types of pain relievers and the pros and cons of each.

Aspirin

Aspirin (brand names: Anacin, Ascriptin, Bayer, Bufferin, Ecotrin, Excedrin) is the most commonly used OTC anti-inflammatory medication. It is cheap and very effective. Sports doctors recommend aspirin to reduce the pain and inflammation seen in the initial stages of most injuries. Aspirin is strong enough to reduce mild to moderate pain caused by inflammation, especially in overuse conditions such as tendinitis (tendon inflammation), neuritis (nerve inflammation), and joint disorders.

Aspirin works by preventing the production of *prostaglandins* that are released when a cell is injured. Imbalances of prostaglandins cause increased local temperature, pain, and inflammation.

The first effects of aspirin are felt in 30 minutes, although its maximum benefits are experienced two hours after the dosage is taken. A slow decline then takes place over the next four to six hours.

Aspirin has well-known side effects. Chief among these is its tendency to irritate the stomach lining, although buffered aspirin helps reduce stomach upsets. Because aspirin thins the blood, it impairs blood clotting and increases the risk of hemorrhage. Prolonged use may cause permanent kidney damage. Also, some people are allergic to aspirin.

Caution must be used when administering aspirin to children who have had recent viral disease (which in some cases can be very mild) because of the link between aspirin use, viral disease, and Reye's syndrome.

Ibuprofen

Ibuprofen (brand names: Advil, Bayer Select Ibuprofen, Midol IB, Motrin IB, Nuprin) is less irritating to the stomach than aspirin and is effective in controlling the pain and inflammation of sports injuries. Only in the last few years has ibuprofen been approved as an OTC drug. Nonmedical personnel frequently recommend ibuprofen for a variety of ailments. This is misguided. While OTC dosages are significantly lower than prescription dosages, ibuprofen is still a powerful drug, and only the amount necessary to reduce symptoms should be used.

Hypothermia and Frostbite

Even on moderately cool days, if a runner's pace becomes too slow or if the weather conditions become cooler during the run, the runner can lose heat faster than it can be produced. Several deaths have been reported due to cold during fun runs, especially in the mountains. Inexperienced marathon runners, who frequently run slower in the second half of the race, are at increased risk of hypothermia, especially on cool, wet, or windy days. Early signs and symptoms of hypothermia are shivering, a false sense of well-being, and an appearance of intoxication. As the body temperature drops further, shivering may stop and excessive drowsiness and muscle weakness may occur. Disorientation, hallucinations, and often a belligerent attitude may follow, and unconsciousness or death is possible.

Injuries caused by cold temperatures are preventable largely through judicious use of protective clothing. On a cool day the clothing worn should consist of multiple thin layers of cotton fibers. A polypropylene fabric may be worn near the skin. This clothing should be covered with an easily removed windbreaker (preferably nylon). As the athlete becomes warm, clothing can be removed to allow sweat to evaporate or dry. However, when the pace gets too slow for the runner to keep warm, the clothes can be put back on.

Appropriate headgear should not be neglected during cold weather since the body loses most of its heat through the head. During wet weather, waterproof breathable clothing is essential.

It is also a good idea to wear sweatsuits while warming up during cool or cold weather. The insulation helps muscles, ligaments, and tendons get warmer and more flexible, which contributes to preventing both acute and overuse injuries.

(continued)

Frostbite

Frostbite is the freezing of skin tissues caused by excessive exposure to cold. Frostbite varies in intensity and is classified according to how deep the freezing penetrates. Mild frostbite, sometimes called "frostnip," is freezing of the superficial layers of skin without blister formation. The characteristic symptoms of mild frostbite are itching, tingling, and numbness. If the condition worsens, the pain begins to abate and may even disappear. Skin also changes color when it is frostbitten. It whitens, then turns red, and finally turns a white purple hue when it is completely frozen. Severe frostbite may involve complete numbness in the area, stiffness, blistering, and in some cases, tissue death that causes gangrene.

The parts of the body at greatest risk of developing frostbite are the tip of the nose, ear lobes and rim, fingertips, and toes.

At the first signs of frostbite, come out of the cold immediately and rewarm the affected area as quickly as possible. The most effective way to thaw frozen skin is to immerse it in a bath kept at a constant temperature of 100 to 105 degrees Fahrenheit for up to an hour. Since rapid rewarming is extremely painful, take two aspirin, ibuprofen, or acetaminophen to relieve the pain.

If there is no access to hot water, put the affected body part under an armpit, between the thighs, or in the groin. If there is the chance the area may refreeze, do not warm it in the first place. If skin has frozen, been rewarmed, then refrozen, the likelihood of damage is drastically increased.

Once the skin has thawed and returned to its normal temperature, bandage the area and seek medical attention at a hospital emergency room. After the doctor has carefully examined the area, he or she will give pain medication and antibiotics, and a tetanus booster if needed. During the following week or weeks, the doctor should monitor the athlete for any signs of infection.

Frostbite can be prevented by wearing proper protection for the face, neck, and extremities during outdoor winter exercise. Winter athletes should wear mutliple layers of lightweight, nonrestrictive clothing.

Acetaminophen

Acetaminophen (brand names: Bayer Select, Excedrin, Midol, Pamprin, Panadol, Tylenol), which does not irritate the stomach, can help reduce pain. However, it does not reduce inflammation. In other words, it controls the symptoms of the inflammation, not the cause.

Naproxin Sodium

Naproxin sodium (brand name: Aleve) has recently been approved for over-the-counter use as an anti-inflammatory and pain reliever. It is a powerful drug and must be used only at the lowest recommended doses.

All OTC anti-inflammatory medications come with labeled directions. Read these carefully. In general, they are taken one at a time with each meal—three a day. Take more only under a doctor's supervision.

When prescribed to treat a sports-related condition, most OTC anti-inflammatory medications are taken in conjunction with using RICE.

Rehabilitating Overuse Running Injuries

Rehabilitation is the process of restoring the injured runner to action by using exercise, therapeutic modalities such as ultrasound and electrical stimulation, and manual therapy (massage and manipulation). Most running injuries can be rehabilitated by runners themselves using exercise alone. In this section we discuss general rehabilitation guidelines for running injuries. Customized rehabilitation prescriptions for individual injuries can be found in chapters 4 through 9.

The three most important goals of the rehabilitation program for overuse running injuries are to

- maintain all-around conditioning,
- establish strength and flexibility in poorly conditioned or imbalanced musculature, and
- reestablish proper running technique.

Maintain All-Around Conditioning

Most runners can maintain their cardiovascular conditioning while injured. For instance, runners with stress fractures of the feet can swim or use stairclimbers, stationary bicycles, cross-country skiing simulators or rowing machines to do cardiovascular exercise.

Remember that lower-body exercise calls into play a larger muscle mass and provides a greater stimulus to the cardiovascular system. Cycling, pool running, stairclimbing, and rowing are preferable to activities such as upper-body ergometry and swimming.

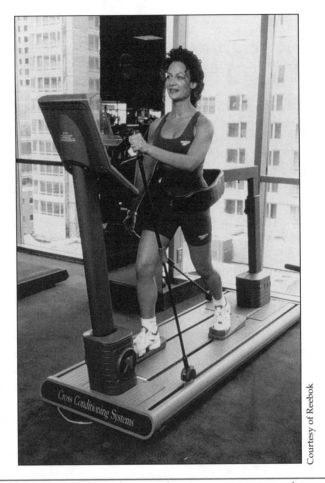

Courtesy of Reebok

Exercise machines are a great way for injured runners to maintain conditioning while avoiding the impact stress of running.

Establish Strength and Flexibility in Poorly Conditioned or Imbalanced Musculature

With allowances made for the injured area, strength and flexibility training should continue as usual. For instance, a runner with a foot ailment can continue to do all upper-body strength and flexibility exercises and can continue to condition the muscles of the hips and thighs.

After mild injuries, strength and flexibility exercises can begin the day after symptoms are first felt, or when there is no local tenderness in the affected area. Even when the injury has deteriorated to the point where symptoms are moderate to severe, exercises should begin within 48 to 72 hours of initiating RICE and OTC medication.

Most overuse running injuries can be rehabilitated by runners themselves using the exercises that appear in chapter 2. Simply adjust the intensity of the exercises to accommodate the limitations of the injury. The more severe the symptoms, the less intense the length of the stretch or the size of the weight used. Never exercise beyond the pain threshold.

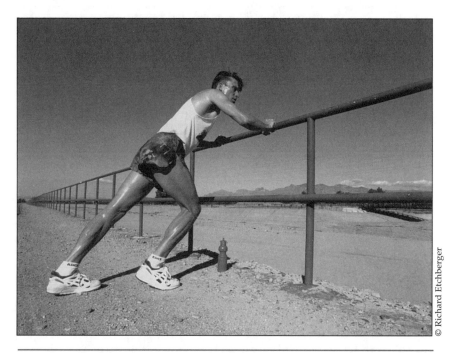

Maintaining flexibility is important to rehabilitation. However, injured runners should adjust the intensity of their exercises and the length of their stretches.

Reestablish Proper Running Technique

After sustaining a severe overuse injury that puts the runner out of action for an extended period, the final step before going back to regular running is to practice running technique.

The original cause of the injury may have been improper technique caused by muscle tightness, especially in the front of the hip (psoas), in back of the thigh (hamstrings), and in the calf and heel cord area in back of the lower leg (gastro-soleus/Achilles tendon unit). Tightness in these areas can interfere with foot strike (see page 8). In such cases, it will only be after the relevant muscle tightness is overcome that proper technique can be restored.

Begin practicing running technique when pain is minimal and there is no limp. Run slowly and on an even surface, focusing on proper technique, especially foot strike. Cut back if it is difficult to maintain proper technique, or if there is pain or swelling.

Heat, Moisture, and the Skin

Prickly heat, or miliaria, frequently affects runners. It primarily affects those who sweat profusely during running. Common symptoms include itching and burning caused by moisture retention in the sweat glands, and a rash of red bumps. The areas commonly affected are the arms, torso, and the creases in the body that allow for bending motions.

Prickly heat is generally not serious but can be highly uncomfortable. Treatment involves bathing the area with hypoallergenic products. The runner should avoid overheating and should not wear constrictive clothing. In general, runners can participate in activities in the heat if they spend sufficient time at rest in a cool, dry area.

Chafing, or intertigo, is another condition extremely common in runners. It begins with a combination of heat and moisture that causes the skin to soften. The friction and repeated rubbing, especially between the thighs, causes the skin to become rubbed raw, or chafed. Chafing describes an area that oozes, then develops lesions that quickly form a crusty, crackling surface.

To treat the affected area, the athlete should use medicated wet packs containing an over-the-counter solution such as Burrows. The area should be treated for approximately 20 minutes, three times a day. Following each treatment, a prescription-strength hydrocortisone cream (1 percent) should be applied topically.

Chafing can be prevented by wearing loose fitting clothing made of natural fibers. Any susceptible areas should be kept as dry and clean as possible during exercise. Male athletes should wear loose cotton boxer shorts under their athletic supporters.

When Is It Necessary to See the Doctor?

If ever in doubt about the symptoms or proper care of an injury, or if self-care measures fail to improve the condition within a reasonable amount of time (two to four weeks), see a doctor. It may also be necessary to see a doctor if an overuse injury has been allowed to become severe, or when symptoms include

- pain before, during, and after running;
- performance affected by pain;
- normal movement affected by pain;
- pain when pressure applied to area;
- swelling; or
- discoloration.

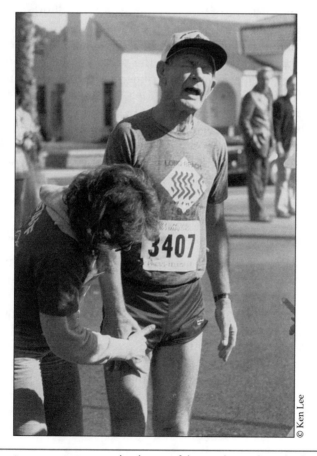

Recurring or intense pain is a good indicator of the need to seek medical attention.

From whom should you seek medical attention? Although the family physician may be qualified to treat certain acute sports injuries such as strains and sprains, he or she may not be the person most capable of treating the overuse injuries seen in runners (although increasingly, primary care physicians are becoming certified in sports medicine). An injured runner should seek the counsel of an orthopedic sports doctor with expertise in running injuries. Such doctors—many of whom are runners themselves—will be sensitive to the special needs of runners and will try to return the runner to full participation quickly and safely. After examining the runner, the doctor may choose to treat the runner him- or herself, or may refer the patient to a therapist or podiatrist.

Doctor-Prescribed Rehabilitation

For overuse injuries, one of the most important contributions the sports doctor can make is to design a rehabilitation program that will correct the runner's condition and return him or her to running with no risk of reinjury. The doctor should initiate the program almost immediately after he or she diagnoses and prescribes treatment for the injury. The notion that treatment and rehabilitation represent two phases of sports injury management is outdated. Treatment and rehabilitation should take place concurrently. The early point at which sports doctors now start rehabilitating injured runners is just one example of how sophisticated the field of rehabilitation has become. Indeed, nowhere in sports medicine has there been more advances than in rehabilitation.

Bites and Stings

Runners often come into contact with stinging insects such as bees, wasps, and hornets. The effects of an attack from one of these insects are usually temporary but painful. Under certain circumstances, however, there may be serious consequences associated with insect stings.

When a bee stings a human, it leaves its stinger and venom sac embedded in its victim's skin and dies shortly thereafter. To prevent more venom from being injected into the skin, remove the stinger and venom sac immediately. Do not try to extract the stinger with fingers or tweezers, as this usually causes more venom to be squirted into the skin. Instead, try to flick out the

(continued)

stinger by quickly scraping a fingernail, knife blade, or credit card over the stinger. Wasps and hornets do not lose their stingers and so they are a continued threat after an attack. After an attack from either a wasp or hornet, leave the area to avoid another attack.

After a bee, wasp, or hornet sting, wash the area with soap and water to prevent bacterial infection (these insects often scavenge in garbage). To reduce pain and swelling, apply cold to the sting, preferably with an ice cube. If ice is not available, a cold can of soda will suffice. Keep applying cold for at least 30 to 45 minutes.

The symptoms of an insect sting may continue for an hour or so. If the pain, swelling, and itching continue for longer than that, take an over-the-counter antihistamine such as diphenhydramine (Benadryl) as label-directed. Aspirin is also an effective means of minimizing swelling and itching.

To help prevent attracting stinging insects, athletes who engage in outdoor sports should avoid scented products like soaps and colognes, as well as brightly colored and very dark clothing.

It is important to note that approximately 1 in 150 people is allergic to bee stings. In these hypersensitive individuals, a bee sting can trigger anaphylactic shock, a severe reaction that can begin within minutes. Symptoms of anaphylactic shock may include the following: nausea; wheezing and difficulty breathing (bronchospasm); cool, clammy, and pale skin; rapid pulse; diarrhea; cramps; extreme thirst; dizziness; and loss of consciousness. If not treated immediately, death may occur.

A warning sign that anaphylactic shock may be developing is swelling in the back of the throat that inhibits breathing and swallowing. Anyone with these symptoms following a bee sting should seek immediate emergency room attention.

A person with a known hypersensitivity to bee stings should seek immediate medical attention when stung. It is recommended that these persons—if they engage in frequent outdoor athletic or recreational activity—carry with them a special emergency kit containing a syringe and the drug epinephrine to counteract the bee venom.

The most important component of rehabilitation for running injuries is an exercise program to promote strength and flexibility in appropriate musculature. In particular, the doctor will identify strength and flexibility imbalances or deficits in the runner and direct a physical therapist to redress these imbalances.

The physical therapist is an indispensable member of the sports medicine team. Physical therapists know exactly which tissues need to be exercised, which exercises are most appropriate to achieve the most effective gains, which equipment is right for different injuries, how hard to push the runner, and when to increase the intensity of the exercise. They know from experience not to push the runner too hard too soon, which can cause reinjury.

Therapeutic exercise is the most effective way to expedite the runner's return to action. A variety of therapeutic modalities have been developed that both promote healing and make exercising more comfortable, and therefore more effective. The traditional therapeutic modalities are ice and heat. During the last quarter century physical therapists have adopted a variety of more high-tech rehabilitation tools, such as ultrasound, electrical stimulation, and traction, to rehabilitate sports injuries.

Almost as important is the emotional support physical therapists provide. They know how tedious and frustrating rehabilitation can be and are trained to motivate runners to continue with rehabilitation.

The physical therapist is also the one, in conjunction with the sports doctor, who okays the patient for return to running after an injury.

It is preferable to be seen by a physical therapist who is experienced in rehabilitating sports injuries. A sports physical therapist will understand the specific physical demands of running. To return the runner to full function, he or she will provide training guidance wherever possible, as well as rehabilitation for the injury itself. Because he or she is treating the person as an athlete, the physical therapist understands that recovery does not just mean overcoming symptoms, but returning to full function. The sports physical therapist must continue treatment until satisfied that it is safe for the runner to return to full participation.

If the athlete finds visits to the doctor's hospital or sports clinic inconvenient, the doctor may refer the person to a physical therapist located closer to where the runner lives or works. Sports physical therapists work in hospitals, in multidisciplinary sports medicine clinics, in physical therapy clinics, or in single-person practices. Student runners, or those engaged in club running, may have their rehabilitation supervised by an athletic trainer.

Foot Injuries

A runner's feet must absorb an enormous amount of stress during training—up to three to four times his or her body weight with each step. Given that runners can take more than 10,000 steps an hour, it is not surprising that these repetitive forces can cause problems in the feet.

Overuse Foot Injuries

Overuse foot injuries include several of the problems seen in other parts of the body, such as stress fractures, tendinitis conditions, bursitis, and irritations of the fascia. Running also brings on a host of unique disorders in the foot. Their prevalence can be explained by the complexity of the foot, the number of anatomical abnormalities associated with it, and the extraordinary stresses to which running subjects it.

An intensive running schedule is often the cause of overuse foot injuries; however, intrinsic factors—poor conditioning, muscle imbalances, or anatomical abnormalities—may be involved. Weakness or tightness in the calf and heel cord area in back of the lower leg may be responsible for plantar fasciitis, an inflammation of the thick band of tissue (the plantar fascia) that runs along the long arch of the foot. Runners with muscle tightness in the front of their hips (psoas muscles), back of the thigh (hamstrings), or the calf and heel cord area in back of the lower leg (gastro-soleus/Achilles tendon unit) tend to have a much briefer-than-normal foot strike because their muscles are so tight they cannot perform the optimal relaxed heel-to-toe foot strike. This improper running technique means that the feet must absorb more stress each time they hit the ground.

Atypical arches are among the most common anatomical abnormalities in the feet that can predispose the athlete to overuse injury. A person with flat feet usually runs with the insides of the feet turned excessively inward. In the feet, this motion, known as pronation, can cause plantar fasciitis and posterior tibial tendinitis. High arches may be responsible for overuse conditions such as heel spurs, Achilles tendinitis, and stress fractures in the foot, lower leg, upper thigh, and pelvis.

An important intrinsic risk factor for overuse foot injuries in women is nutritional abuse. This risk factor is associated exclusively with the occurrence of stress fractures in women who may be suffering bone density loss due to irregular menstruation—generally a result of an eating disorder. When exposed to the repetitive demands of exercise such as jogging or aerobics, bones in the foot and lower leg are susceptible to stress fractures. For more information on the predisposition of some female runners to stress fractures, see chapter 10.

How Do Stress Fractures Occur?

A stress fracture is a series of microfractures caused by repetitive, low-grade trauma in activities such as running, dancing, and aerobics. Two theories have been proposed to explain how stress fractures develop.

1. Fatigue theory: When tired, the muscles cannot support the skeleton as well as they can when they are not tired. Running activities that exhaust the muscles therefore increase the load on the bones. When its tolerance is exceeded, tiny cracks appear in the bone's surface.

2. Overload theory: Muscles contract in such a way that they pull on the bone. For instance, the contraction of the calf muscles bends the tibia forward like a drawn bow. The backward and forward bending of the bone can cause cracks to appear in the front of the tibia.

When the stress fracture takes place in the tibia, it occurs in the top two-thirds of that bone. In the fibula, stress fractures usually take place two or three inches above the lateral malleolus (the outer ankle bone).

Thinner bones are at greater risk of sustaining stress fractures. Because one of the side effects of irregular menstruation is bone thinning, girls and women with eating disorders and menstrual irregularities are at greater risk of these overuse injuries. For much more on the relationship between eating disorders, menstrual irregularities, and stress fractures, refer to the chapter "Special Concerns for Female Runners."

Extrinsic factors affecting overuse foot injuries usually involve training errors, inappropriate workout structure, and improper footwear. (For a general discussion of intrinsic and extrinsic risk factors involved in overuse running injuries, see chapter 1; injury prevention guidelines can be found in chapter 2.)

STRESS FRACTURES OF THE HEEL BONE, NAVICULAR BONE, AND LONG BONES OF THE MIDFOOT

Foot

(A series of microfractures that develop in one or more of the bones in the foot, usually the long bones of the midfoot, the metatarsals.)

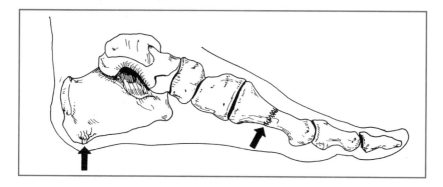

If you have distinct pain in one or more of the foot bones, you may have a stress fracture. Stress fractures are caused by repetitive low-intensity impact to the foot bones. Diagnosing stress fractures may be quite difficult not only because the onset of symptoms is so gradual, but because X rays do not reveal the stress fracture until three to six weeks after the symptoms first occur (in medical terms, they are occult).

An intensive running schedule often precipitates stress fractures, though they are more likely to occur if one or more of the following risk factors exist:

INTRINSIC   Anatomical abnormalities—High arches, flat feet, shorter-than-normal first metatarsal bone (Morton's foot), bunions.

Poor conditioning or muscle imbalances—Tight muscles in the front of the hip (psoas), back of the thigh (hamstrings), back of the lower leg (gastro-soleus/Achilles tendon unit), and the area on the underside of the foot (plantar fascia).

Nutritional abuse—Women who menstruate irregularly because of poor diet and excessive exercise often develop bone thinning and are therefore at increased risk of stress fractures.

Incorrect running technique—A briefer-than-optimal foot strike means the feet have to absorb excessive stress each time they hit the ground, which may cause injuries in the feet; tightness in certain muscle groups may interfere with optimum foot strike.

EXTRINSIC Training errors—Rapid increases in the frequency, intensity, or duration of the running regimen.

Improper footwear—Worn-out shoes, shoes with inadequate arch support, shoes with an excessively stiff sole.

Symptoms:

- Onset of symptoms is gradual.
- Pain is felt in the affected bone during activity.
- Distinct pain and swelling occur over the affected bone.

Concerns:

- If allowed to worsen, a complete displaced fracture may occur.

Treatment:

What you can do

- Suspend running schedule, but do not completely discontinue exercise (see "Rehabilitation").
- Ice massage the area of pain.
- For relief of minor to moderate pain, take acetaminophen or ibuprofen as label-directed, or for the relief of pain *and* inflammation, take aspirin if tolerated.
- Use a doughnut pad to relieve pressure on the area.
- If the pain is severe, or if it does not clear up in two weeks, consult a sports doctor.

What the doctor can do

- The doctor will probably take X rays to confirm the diagnosis. If the X rays are negative, as they are in half of all cases (stress fractures do not show up until three to six weeks after symptoms are first felt), the doctor may take another set of X rays two weeks later. If the X rays are negative, and a stress fracture is suspected, a bone scan may be taken.
- If the stress fracture is severe, the doctor may protect the injured foot by prescribing a removable cast for several weeks to prevent further stress.
- Depending on the underlying cause of the stress fracture, the doctor may prescribe anti-inflammatory medication, orthotics (if the patient has flat feet or high arches), physical therapy (if the patient has tight Achilles tendons), more appropriate footwear (if the athlete's footwear is to blame), or nutritional counseling (if the patient is female and experiencing menstrual irregularities).

Rehabilitation:

- Engage in nonweightbearing cardiovascular exercise that does not aggravate the condition, such as swimming and stationary biking, and, making allowances for the injured area, continue as usual with strength and flexibility conditioning.
- Engage in a flexibility program for the entire lower extremities. If pain persists for more than two weeks, consult a certified sports doctor (see pages 83-86). The doctor should prescribe an exercise program to alleviate muscle imbalances or strength and flexibility deficits that may be the underlying causes of the condition. The rehabilitation exercises may be supervised by a physical therapist or done independently. Particular attention should be paid to stretching and strengthening the muscles in the lower leg. Also, if it is determined that the runner has tightness in certain muscle groups that may interfere with running form, such as in the muscles in the front of the hip (psoas), in back of the thigh (hamstrings), and the calf and heel cord area in back of the lower leg (gastro-soleus/Achilles tendon unit), stretching should be done in those areas.

Return to running:

- Resume running six to eight weeks after the onset of treatment and rehabilitation, or when symptoms have gone.

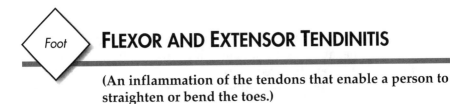

FLEXOR AND EXTENSOR TENDINITIS

(An inflammation of the tendons that enable a person to straighten or bend the toes.)

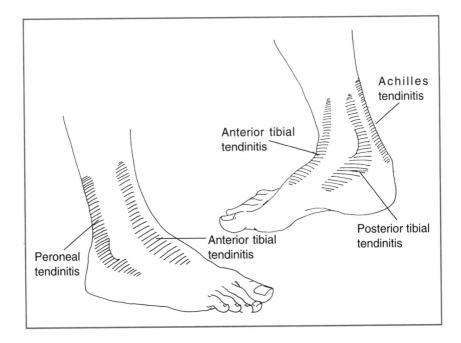

If you have pain, a creaking sensation (crepitus), and puffy swelling on top of one or more of your feet, and the symptoms intensify when running and either bending or straightening your toes, you may have flexor or extensor tendinitis.

An intensive running schedule usually precipitates flexor tendinitis or extensor tendinitis, though it is more likely to occur if the following risk factor exists:

EXTRINSIC Improper footwear—Shoes that are laced too tightly, causing pressure on the tendons from the tongue of the shoe.

Symptoms:

- Onset of symptoms is gradual.
- Pain and puffy swelling occur on top of the foot. Pain intensifies when either bending or straightening the toes, especially when running. Pain is elicited by pressing the affected toes.
- In severe cases the runner feels a creaking sensation (crepitus).
- The runner may walk with a limp.

Concerns:

- Tendons are notoriously slow healers, and if the condition is allowed to deteriorate, it can be difficult to overcome.

Treatment:

What you can do

- For the first 48 to 72 hours, administer ice massage and reduce stress on the affected tendons by suspending your running schedule and not wearing shoes. When you must wear shoes (1) loosen the laces so the tongue does not compress the top of the foot, (2) place a foam rubber pad with a gap cut in it on top of the foot to keep direct pressure off the tendons, and (3) tie the laces in a stepladder fashion, not crisscross.
- For relief of minor to moderate pain, take acetaminophen or ibuprofen as label-directed, or for the relief of pain *and* inflammation, take aspirin if tolerated.
- Almost always, the above self-treatment will resolve the condition.
- If the condition persists for more than two weeks, consult a sports doctor.

What the doctor can do

- If the above treatment has not or does not work under the doctor's supervision, the doctor may administer a cortisone injection into the area around the tendon. Such an injection should be followed by two weeks of complete rest from running or strenuous activities using the foot.

Rehabilitation:

- Engage in cardiovascular exercise that does not involve repetitive downward bending of the foot (such as using a rowing machine) and, making allowances for the injured area, continue as usual with strength and flexibility conditioning.

- Engage in a flexibility program for the entire lower extremities. If pain persists for more than two weeks, consult a certified sports doctor (see pages 83-86). The doctor should prescribe an exercise program to alleviate muscle imbalances or strength and flexibility deficits that may be the underlying causes of the condition. The rehabilitation exercises may be supervised by a physical therapist or done independently. Particular attention should be paid to stretching the muscles and tendons of the calf and heel cord area in back of the lower leg (gastro-soleus/Achilles tendon unit), and strengthening the muscles in the foot itself that are responsible for bending and straightening the toes.

Return to running:

- Resume running two weeks after the onset of treatment and rehabilitation, or when symptoms have gone.

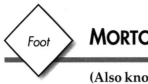

MORTON'S NEUROMA

(Also known as interdigital neuroma or plantar neuroma, a nerve inflammation in the foot caused by the nerve being pinched between the third and fourth toes or, less often, between the second and third toes.)

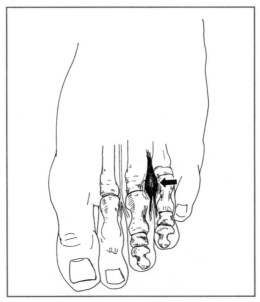

If you have recurrent pain from the outside of one toe to the inner side of the adjoining one (usually between the third and fourth toes), as well as radiating pain and numbness in the affected toes, you may have a condition known as Morton's neuroma, sometimes called an interdigital neuroma or a plantar neuroma.

An intensive running schedule usually precipitates a neuroma in the foot, though it is more likely to occur if one or more of the following risk factors exist:

INTRINSIC   Anatomical abnormalities—Unusually large bony prominences in the joints of the midfoot.

EXTRINSIC   Improper footwear—Running shoes that are too narrow.

Symptoms:

- Onset of symptoms is gradual.
- There is recurrent pain from the outer side of one toe to the inner side of the adjoining one. Usually the pain occurs between the third and fourth toes.
- The pain worsens when tight shoes are worn and may go away entirely when the runner is barefoot.
- The pain is often described as resembling a mild electric shock.
- There is often radiating pain and numbness in the affected toes. These symptoms can be triggered by squeezing the ball of the foot between the affected metatarsals.

Concerns:

Unless treated, the condition can result in persistent pain.

Treatment:

What you can do

- For 48 to 72 hours after symptoms are first felt, administer ice massage and reduce stress on the inflamed nerve by suspending your running schedule (but do not completely discontinue exercise—see "Rehabilitation"), wearing wider, softer shoes that do not compress the bones, and wearing a foam rubber pad in the shoe below the ball of the affected foot.
- For relief of minor to moderate pain, take acetaminophen or ibuprofen as label-directed, or for the relief of pain *and* inflammation, take aspirin if tolerated.

- If the condition does not clear up, or if it clears up and then recurs, consult a sports doctor.

What the doctor can do

- If the athlete has followed the above treatment regimen, and the symptoms do not abate, or if they resolve and then recur, the doctor may prescribe anti-inflammatories, a cortisone injection, or a metatarsal bar (a special shoe insert or orthotic that helps spread apart the bones pinching the nerve).
- If pain and limp persist despite the above techniques, surgery may be necessary. During the procedure the nerve is removed. The patient is left with no sensation in the affected toes, but most contend this is preferable to the pain. After surgery, the athlete wears a dressing for three weeks and a postoperative shoe with a firm sole.

Rehabilitation:

- Engage in nonweightbearing cardiovascular exercise that does not aggravate the condition, such as swimming and stationary biking, and, making allowances for the injured area, continue as usual with strength and flexibility conditioning.
- Engage in a flexibility program for the entire lower extremities. If pain persists for more than two weeks, consult a certified sports doctor (see pages 83-86). The doctor should prescribe an exercise program to alleviate muscle imbalances or strength and flexibility deficits that may be the underlying causes of the condition. The rehabilitation exercises may be supervised by a physical therapist or done independently. Particular attention should be paid to stretching the band of tissue that runs along the underside of the foot (plantar fascia) and the muscles and tendons of the calf and heel cord area in back of the lower leg (gastro-soleus/Achilles tendon unit).

Return to running:

- Resume running two weeks after the onset of treatment and rehabilitation, or when symptoms have gone.

Recovery time:

- If surgery is necessary, go back to running six weeks after the operation or as advised by your doctor.

SESAMOIDITIS

Foot

(An inflammation of one of the oval-shaped sesamoid bones that lie within one of the tendons in the foot, usu- ally affecting one or both of the sesamoids underneath the long bone that connects to the big toe.)

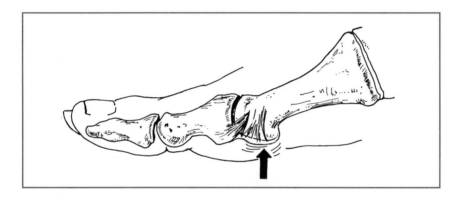

If you have pain in the fleshy ball of your foot just behind the big toe, which may extend to the arch, and this pain becomes especially acute during the toe-off phase of the running cycle, you may have sesamoidi- tis.

Sesamoiditis is caused by repetitive, low-intensity stress experienced by the sesamoids during the toe-off stage of the running cycle. An inten- sive running schedule usually precipitates this condition.

Symptoms:

- Onset of symptoms is gradual.
- Pain is felt on the fleshy ball of the foot just behind the big toe, which may extend into the arch. Pain is especially acute during the toe-off phase of the running cycle. The big toe is usually stiff and weak.

Concerns:

- If allowed to deteriorate, the sesamoid may fracture completely, may "die" because of interrupted blood supply, or may develop arthritis.

Treatment:

What you can do

- Suspend running schedule, but do not completely discontinue exercise (see "Rehabilitation").
- Wear a quarter-inch-thick foam pad under the sesamoids when returning to running. To make the pad, obtain a piece of foam rubber from a pharmacy, trim it so it is two inches long and one and a half inches wide, and affix it in place with adhesive tape or "sticky spray" such as tincture of benzoin (available in most pharmacies).
- Stretch the toes each time before exercising.
- For relief of minor to moderate pain, take acetaminophen or ibuprofen as label-directed, or for the relief of pain *and* inflammation, take aspirin if tolerated.
- If the condition persists for more than two weeks, consult a sports doctor.

What the doctor can do

- If the above measures fail, the doctor may prescribe anti-inflammatories, cortisone injections (a series of three injections may be necessary), or a shoe insert that prevents the big toe from bending upward.
- If the doctor's treatment fails, surgery may be done to remove the sesamoid, although this is rarely necessary.

Rehabilitation:

- Engage in cardiovascular exercise such as stationary biking (wear a shoe with a rigid sole and exert pressure with the middle part of the foot), and, making allowances for the injured area, continue as usual with strength and flexibility conditioning.
- Engage in a flexibility program for the entire lower extremities. If pain persists for more than two weeks, consult a certified sports doctor (see pages 83-86). The doctor should prescribe an exercise program to alleviate muscle imbalances or strength and flexibility deficits that may be the underlying causes of the condition. The rehabilitation exercises may be supervised by a physical therapist or done independently. Particular attention should be paid to stretching the band of tissue that runs along the underside of the foot (plantar fascia) and the muscles and tendons of the calf and heel cord area in back of the lower leg (gastro-soleus/Achilles tendon unit), and strengthening the muscles in the lower leg that

control upward bending, or dorsiflexion, of the foot (tibialis anterior, flexor tibialis posterior, flexor digitorum longus, flexor hallucis longus).

Recovery time:

- This condition may clear up within four to six weeks or may not clear up at all unless surgery is done.

BUNIONS

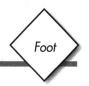

Foot

(A deformity of the big toe that causes it to angle outward by more than 10 to 15 degrees so that the tip of the toe points toward the smaller toes. A bunionette is the same condition but it affects the little toe.)

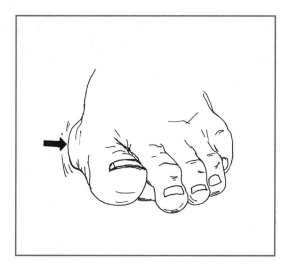

If your big toe angles outward so that its tip points inward toward the smaller toes, and you have pain over the bony prominence, you may have a bunion.

Bunions are usually congenital or genetic, though they may be brought on by an intensive running schedule in association with the following risk factors:

INTRINSIC Anatomical abnormalities—Flat feet (the exaggerated rolling-in action created when running exerts an angular push on the big toe).

EXTRINSIC Improper footwear—Tight-fitting high-heeled shoes (bunions are seen more often in women).

Symptoms:

- The big toe is angled outward by an angle greater than 10 to 15 degrees; the tip of the toe points inward toward the smaller toes.
- Pain is felt directly over the bunion, and the area may look red and inflammed.
- A callus may develop on the sole of the foot behind the second toe.

Concerns:

- When allowed to deteriorate, friction from running shoes or daily footwear can cause a growth of cartilage and bone (exostosis) to develop over the bone where the angle is greatest. A bursitis can develop over the exostosis, which itself can cause great pain.
- As a consequence of the second toe sliding under the angled big toe, a separate but related condition known as "hammertoe" can develop (see pages 101-103).

Treatment:

What you can do

- Wear wider running shoes, and wider, softer shoes during daily activities.
- Use ice, compression, and elevation after running or other intensive weightbearing activity.
- Use a toe spacer to straighten the big toe and reduce the likelihood of hammertoe in the second toe, wear a doughnut pad over the outside of the bony prominence on the side of the big toe to reduce friction, or cut a hole in the running shoe near the bunion to give the bunion more room.
- For relief of minor to moderate pain, take acetaminophen or ibuprofen as label-directed, or for the relief of pain *and* inflammation, take aspirin if tolerated.
- If running becomes difficult, consult a sports doctor.

What the doctor can do

- If self-treatment measures do not work, the doctor may recommend or prescribe anti-inflammatories, orthotics (if flat feet are responsible for the condition), or shoes that do not aggravate the condition.
- In many cases, surgery may be required to enable pain-free running. This procedure involves cutting into the first metatarsal, straightening it, and then pinning it in place.

Rehabilitation:

- No rehabilitation program exists to correct this condition, other than stretching the toe _away_ from the bunion (down and inside), and strengthening the foot muscles that enable a person to force his big toe sideways. Continue with running schedule unless pain makes this impossible.

Recovery time:

- Symptoms may diminish if the appropriate measures are taken, but the bunion itself will usually not straighten unless surgery is done.

HAMMERTOE

Foot

(A buckling-under of the end of the second toe, which may eventually become permanent.)

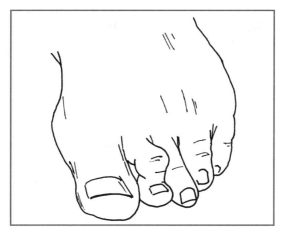

If your second toe is buckled under, and you have pain at the tip of the toe where it comes into contact with the inside of the shoe and a hard corn or callus on top of the toe, you may have a hammertoe.

Hammertoe is caused by the repetitive bumping of the second toe against the inside front of the running shoe.

This condition is usually congenital or genetic, though it may be brought on by an intensive running schedule in association with one or more of the following risk factors:

INTRINSIC   Anatomical abnormalities—Flat front arch or bunions (which cause the deformed big toe to slide under the second toe when the forefoot is compressed by shoes, thereby lifting it and causing it to bump against the inside of the shoe).

EXTRINSIC   Improper footwear—Shoes or running shoes that are too tight or too narrow (thus women are at greater risk of developing a hammertoe).

Symptoms:

- Pain is felt at the tip of the toe where it comes in contact with the inside of the front of the shoe.
- The toe is usually buckled under.
- Due to friction, a callus or hard corn usually forms on the top of the toe.
- The top of the toe is often red and inflamed.

Concerns:

- If allowed to deteriorate, the tendons under the toe become very tight while at the same time the tendons on top of the toe loosen, which makes it very difficult for the toe to return to its normal shape without resorting to surgery.

Treatment:

What you can do

- Wear shoes and running shoes of proper length and width.
- Apply a doughnut pad to the top of the affected toe or toes to reduce friction and irritation.
- Stretch out the toes often. Tape the toes to maintain their symmetry.

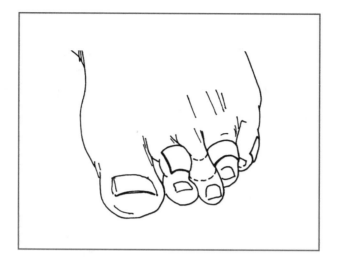

- For relief of minor to moderate pain, take acetaminophen or ibuprofen as label-directed, or for the relief of pain *and* inflammation, take aspirin if tolerated.
- If pain makes running difficult, consult a sports doctor.

What the doctor can do

- If the above measures do not succeed, surgery may be necessary. In this procedure, the flexor tendon is severed so the toe can straighten, and the toe is cut and kept in a straightened position with a wire. After the operation, the foot is bandaged for three weeks, during which time a wooden-soled shoe is worn to protect the wound. Three weeks later the stitches are removed, and for six weeks thereafter, the toe is taped so it is bent slightly upward.

Rehabilitation:

- Other than stretching the muscles in the foot that provide for toe extension (upward turning) and strengthening the muscles that facilitate toe flexion (downward turning), no rehabilitation program exists to correct this condition. Continue with running schedule unless pain makes this impossible.

Recovery time:

- Running can begin six to twelve weeks after surgery.

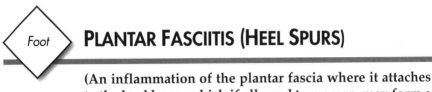

Foot ▸ PLANTAR FASCIITIS (HEEL SPURS)

(An inflammation of the plantar fascia where it attaches
to the heel bone, which if allowed to worsen, may form a
bone spur.)

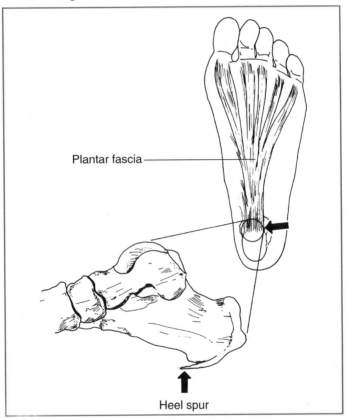

Plantar fascia

Heel spur

If you have pain and tenderness on the inner side of the sole of your foot,
just in front of the heel, you may have plantar fasciitis. This condition is
caused by repetitive stretching of the plantar fascia when the runner lifts
the heel during the push-off stage of the stride.

An intensive running schedule may precipitate plantar fasciitis, though
it is more likely to occur if one or more of the following risk factors exist:

INTRINSIC   Anatomical abnormalities—Flat feet, high arches,
             knock knees, or feet that pronate (turn inward)
             when running.

Poor conditioning or muscle imbalances—Tight, inflexible calf muscles or Achilles tendons.

Incorrect running technique—A briefer-than-optimal foot strike means the feet have to absorb excessive stress each time they hit the ground, which may cause injuries in the feet; such a foot strike may be caused by tightness in certain muscle groups.

EXTRINSIC   Footwear—Worn-out shoes, shoes with inadequate arch support, shoes with an excessively stiff sole.

Training schedule—Rapid increase in frequency, intensity, or duration of running regimen.

Symptoms:

- Pain or tenderness is felt on the inner side of the sole, immediately in front of the fleshy part of the heel.
- Symptoms are especially intense early in the day; they may gradually diminish, and then reintensify with increased weightbearing activity.
- The person tends to avoid walking on the heel, favoring forefoot instead.
- Symptoms intensify when walking on heels or tiptoes.
- In severe cases, numbness develops on the outside of the foot.

Treatment:

What you can do

- For the first 48 to 72 hours, administer ice massage and reduce stress on the plantar fascia by suspending running schedule, wearing one-eighth-inch heel wedge in shoe (or "heel cups," available in most pharmacies), and avoid walking in bare feet.
- Continue cardiovascular activities that do not involve weightbearing—swimming and stationary biking are especially beneficial. After the initial symptoms abate, start gentle stretching of the calf muscle/Achilles tendon unit and the plantar fascia.
- When there is no tenderness, no limp, and no pain in the morning (this may take six weeks), *gradually* return to running, ideally on a forgiving surface such as grass or dirt.
- If any of the anatomical abnormalities or strength or flexibility deficits described above are suspected, or if the symptoms persist for longer than six weeks despite following the above treatment program, consult a sports doctor.

What the doctor can do

- Depending on the underlying cause of the condition, the doctor may prescribe anti-inflammatory medication, orthotics (if the patient has flat feet or knock knees), physical therapy (if the patient has tight calf muscles or Achilles tendons), or steroid injections.
- If these measures do not succeed in correcting the condition within four to six months, or if bone spurs have developed, surgery may be necessary.

Rehabilitation:

- Engage in cardiovascular exercise that does not aggravate the condition, such as swimming and cycling, and, making allowances for the injured area, continue as usual with strength and flexibility conditioning.
- Engage in a flexibility program for the entire lower extremities. If pain persists for more than two weeks, consult a certified sports doctor (see pages 83-86). The doctor should prescribe an exercise program to alleviate muscle imbalances or strength and flexibility deficits that may be the underlying causes of the condition. The rehabilitation exercises may be supervised by a physical therapist or done independently. Particular attention should be paid to stretching the plantar fascia itself, as well as the muscles and tendons of the calf and heel cord area in back of the lower leg (gastrosoleus/Achilles tendon unit), and strengthening the muscles in the lower leg that control upward bending, or dorsiflexion, of the foot (tibialis anterior, flexor tibialis posterior, flexor digitorum longus, flexor hallucis longus).

Recovery time:

- Even when plantar fasciitis is caught in its early stages, at least six weeks of relative rest is usually necessary before the foot has no pain and the person can return to running.
- Chronic plantar fasciitis may take several months to a year to clear up, and sometimes it may not clear up at all unless surgery is done.

Nonorthopedic Foot Problems

Risk factors such as wearing inappropriate footwear and anatomical abnormalities may also play a role in causing nonorthopedic foot problems. Although these problems may be less severe than overuse foot injuries, they nonetheless can cause a runner great distress and affect running technique and training schedules.

Blisters

Blisters are portions of the skin that become irritated due to friction, causing them to fill up with clear fluid, blood, or pus. They can be extremely disabling, especially when they open. They frequently occur in the foot, especially the ball of the foot and the heel.

Blisters commonly affect runners at the beginning of the season, after a long layoff, when beginning a running program, or when breaking in a new pair of running shoes.

To prevent blisters that may occur in the above circumstances, dust the skin with talcum powder or apply petroleum jelly (such as Vaseline). Wearing two pairs of socks also helps reduce friction and is especially helpful to the runner who has sensitive skin or sweats excessively. Certain types of socks have special reinforcement in high-risk areas to reduce friction. Thorlo, for instance, makes socks to accommodate the frictional forces exerted in twelve sports. The extra padding also helps protect against stress fractures.

If a sore spot occurs, the runner should cover the area with a friction-reducing substance such as petroleum jelly or moleskin (available at most pharmacies).

If a blister does develop, the runner should remember the very real potential for serious infection if the blister is mismanaged. A doctor should see any blister that becomes infected.

Keep the surface of the blister intact because it acts as a protective barrier against bacteria. It is usually unwise to deliberately break a blister. Instead, wear a doughnut pad to protect it against further friction.

It may be necessary to preemptively break a blister if it is likely to tear itself. In such cases, sterilize a needle by holding it over a flame until it turns red hot. Let it cool and then pierce the skin just inside the edge of the blister. The blister should be opened wide enough so that it does not reseal. After the fluid has dispersed, place a pressure pad over the blister to prevent it from refilling with fluid. After five or six days, the skin should have hardened and can be cut away.

Always choose the nonaggressive method of treating blisters to reduce the potential for infection. A blister that tears by itself should be cared for as follows:

- Clean the area with soap and water, then rinse with an antiseptic.
- Using sterile scissors, cut the torn blister halfway around its perimeter so there is a ring of blistered skin around its edge.

- Apply antiseptic and a mild ointment such as zinc oxide to the exposed tissue.
- Lay the cutoff flap of skin over the exposed tissue and cover the area with a sterile dressing.
- Within two or three days, the underlying skin should have hardened sufficiently, and the dead skin can be removed.
- The runner should wear a Band-Aid for a week afterward.

Corns

There are two types of corns: hard and soft.

Hard corns (clavis durum) are thick nodules of skin that usually develop over the middle joint of the second or third toe. They are caused by the friction created by rubbing inside the shoes, often as a result of too-narrow shoes that cause the second and third toes to buckle. Hard corns are often seen in runners with hammertoe (see pages 101-103). The runner can alleviate symptoms by soaking the foot daily in warm soapy water to soften the skin, wearing properly fitting shoes, and wearing a doughnut pad over the corn. However, if the underlying cause of the corn is a hammertoe, that troublesome condition will have to be corrected before the corn will go away.

A combination of wearing too-narrow shoes and profuse sweating is usually the cause of soft corns (clavi molle). This type of corn usually develops between the fourth and fifth toes. These small, conical-shaped growths create pain because the skin on top of the corn is always flaking, leaving a tender portion of skin underneath. To treat soft corns, wear wider shoes, keep the skin between the toes clean and dry, wear a corn pad between the toes, and apply 40 percent salicyclic acid (available at pharmacies in liquid or patch form).

Calluses

A callus is a thickening of the skin caused by repetitive friction. Pain is caused by the loss of elasticity in the skin and the tightness in the running shoes created by the thickened skin. Calluses may be caused by too-tight or too-narrow running shoes, or by an anatomical abnormality such as bunions or bunionettes, hammer- or claw toes, or flat feet—conditions that cause the foot or the way it moves to exert increased pressure and friction inside the shoe.

In the foot, the most common sites of calluses are the heel, the ball of the foot, the top of the hammer- or claw toes, and the inner side of the big toe.

The runner can prevent calluses by wearing two pairs of socks (a thin cotton or nylon pair next to the skin, a heavy athletic pair over those) or double-knit socks. Socks made with reinforcement in high-risk areas reduce friction.

In the initial stages, anyone who develops a callus should file it with an emery file after showering. Massaging small amounts of lanolin into the softened skin may help maintain elasticity.

Once a thick callus has formed, use a keratolytic agent such as Whitehead's ointment. Salicylic acid, 5 to 10 percent strength (available at pharmacies), can be applied at night and peeled off in the morning.

If the callus does not go away and causes pain, make an appointment to see a chiropodist, who may remove the excess skin by sanding, pumicing, or paring it off with a sharp knife.

Warts or Verrucae

Warts, or verrucae as they are sometimes called, are caused by a virus that is often transmitted from one athlete to another by the floor of showers and locker rooms or anywhere people walk barefoot.

They are usually located on the sole of the foot, are round or oval-shaped, and have a crack or dark spot in the middle. This distinctive mark distinguishes warts from calluses or corns.

Warts are susceptible to infection, especially on the sole of the foot, where they are constantly irritated. The runner should prevent this irritation by using a doughnut pad.

After a hot foot bath, file down the wart as far as possible with an emery board; then treat it with an over-the-counter wart ointment. This may have to be continued for several months before the wart goes away.

If the pain is severe, it may be preferable to see a podiatrist, who will cut or burn away the wart.

Athlete's Foot (Tinea Pedis)

Athlete's foot is a fungus that causes the skin between the toes to become soggy, cracked, scaly, and chalky-looking. The soles of the affected feet and toes become extremely itchy. Feet that develop this condition often smell offensive.

The cause of athlete's foot is poor foot hygiene and not drying the feet thoroughly after showers or baths. Because the condition is contagious, it is relatively common in runners who spend time walking barefoot on damp locker room floors.

Since athlete's foot is a troublesome condition to overcome, the focus should be on prevention:

- Wash the feet regularly with soap and water, dry them thoroughly after showering or bathing, and use talcum powder on the feet.
- Always wear clean socks and change them daily.
- Wear porous running shoes that allow air circulation and evaporation of moisture.
- Wear slippers or flip flops when walking around locker rooms.

If athlete's foot develops, follow the above steps and use a standard over-the-counter fungicide as label-directed. Brand names include Resenex and Tinactin.

If the condition does not clear up in two weeks, seek medical treatment from the family doctor or a podiatrist.

Ingrown Toenails

An ingrown toenail describes a condition in which the edges of a toenail grow in such a way that they dig into the surrounding skin. This condition usually affects the big toe. Ingrown toenails may be caused by tight-fitting shoes or improper care of the nails.

To prevent ingrown toenails, wear shoes that fit comfortably and cut the nails at least once a week, making sure to cut the nail straight across so the sharp edges of the nail do not grow into the surrounding skin.

If an ingrown toenail develops, see a chiropodist, who may use surgical or nonsurgical measures to correct the condition. Keep in mind that infections can easily develop in an ingrown toenail.

Black Nails (Subungual Hematoma)

Repetitive impact to the front of the big toe can cause blood to form under the nail. It is usually seen in runners who wear shoes that are too small or who run downhill a lot, which causes the nail to be pried upward with each step. When the nail becomes separated from the underlying tissue, pain develops under the nail, where a pooling of blood can be seen. Often, the nail falls off.

The most important measure is to wear shoes that provide the big toe with enough room to move, and to avoid running downhill too much. It may be helpful to wear padding over the nail to prevent it from being pried upward.

If the condition is painful, see a doctor, who may relieve the condition by sterilizing a tool (such as a paper clip) over a flame until it glows red, letting it cool down, and then passing the hot end through the nail, allowing blood to escape and thus relieving pressure on the nail.

5

Ankle Injuries

Running places extraordinary repetitive stresses on the ankle joint, so it is a logical site of injury. The ankle is also the site of one of the very few acute injuries sustained by runners—the ankle sprain. (An acute injury is one that occurs suddenly as a result of significant stress; overuse injuries develop over time from repetitive low-intensity stress to tissues.) Due to the relatively high incidence of ankle sprains in runners, this acute injury merits special attention. Overuse ankle injuries will be covered later.

Ankle Sprains

Ankle sprains are usually caused by the runner taking a misstep on an uneven running surface. Most doctors consider the ankle sprain to be among the most common acute sports injuries. Yet ankle sprains get little respect, despite the fact that they can cause chronic instability in the ankle. Even mild ankle sprains must be treated seriously.

In recent years there have been major advances in the way ankle sprains are treated, characterized by early range of motion as opposed to lengthy immobilization. This aggressive attitude toward treating ankle sprains should be of interest to all athletes, runners included, given the frequency with which this injury occurs.

Ankle sprains are usually caused by a *twist* of the ankle. An ankle that sprains because the runner rolls over on the outside of the ankle is an *inversion* sprain; sprains caused by turn-ins are *eversion* sprains.

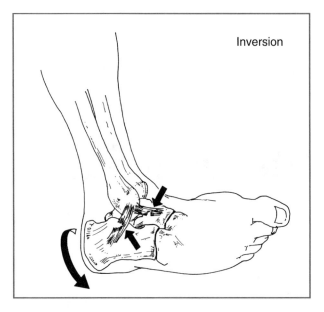

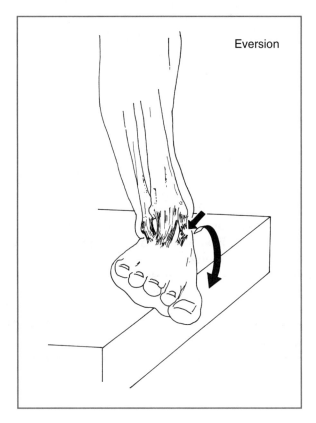

Inversion sprains are much more common than eversion sprains. That is because there is more bony stability on the outer side of the ankle, which makes the inner side of the ankle more likely to give way. This allows the outer side to roll over and cause stretches or tears of the ligament on that side.

Usually one or two ligaments are sprained. If only one ligament is sprained, it is usually the anterior talofibular ligament, but if the ankle bends over farther, the calcaneal fibular ligament may also be injured.

Eversion ankle sprains are seen less frequently. These kinds of sprains usually occur when the runner steps into a hole and the ankle simultaneously bends inward and rotates outward. Usually the damage takes place in the anterior talofibular ligament, the interosseus ligament, or the deltoid ligament. Unless treated properly, the instability created by an eversion ankle sprain can cause degeneration in the talus, which may in turn lead to the onset of arthritis.

As with all sprains, ankle sprains are classified according to their severity—first, second, or third degree. Instability is one of the characteristic symptoms of an ankle sprain, and testing instability is one of the most important means of judging how badly sprained the ankle is. Remember that the swelling that quickly takes place may cause the joint to stiffen, thereby disguising the instability and perhaps leading to a misdiagnosis as a first-degree sprain. Therefore, the sooner a doctor examines the ankle injury, the more accurate the diagnosis.

Acute ankle injuries are often caused by freak accidents—tripping in a rut, for instance—and may be difficult to prevent. There are several preventive measures, however, that runners can take to avoid acute ankle injuries.

Most important, runners should engage in a conditioning program to develop strength and flexibility in the tissues around the ankle joint. Flexibility in the Achilles tendon is of particular importance. An ankle that can bend upward at least 15 degrees can more efficiently accommodate the forces that cause ankle sprains than an ankle with less flexibility. All athletes should stretch their Achilles tendons before exercise, and those with naturally tight Achilles tendons should place extra emphasis on stretching this area. Strength and flexibility should also be developed in all the muscle-tendon units of the lower leg.

Strength in the peroneal muscles (those in the front, outer side of the lower leg) are especially important to prevent rolling over on the ankle and sustaining an inversion sprain.

Wearing appropriate footwear is another important way of preventing acute ankle injuries. Runners should run in footwear specifically designed for running. At the same time, runners should not participate in other sports while wearing their running shoes. For instance, running shoes should not be worn to play tennis or do aerobics, two sports with high demands for side-to-side movements.

After an acute ankle injury such as a sprain, a person often loses proprioceptive skills—the ability to know what different parts of the body are doing without looking at them. Coordination between the ankle and foot suffers the most, which can lead to further sprains. After sustaining a sprain, it is important for the runner to regain proprioception by using a device such as a "wobble-board."

Traditionally, runners used tape to protect the ankle from reinjury. Applying tape was time consuming and required the help of a skilled person. Most runners these days use ready-made braces to prevent reinjury. These braces should not be used *in place* of conditioning, but may be helpful *in conjunction* with conditioning.

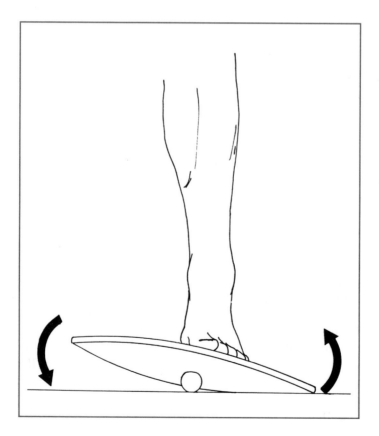

ANKLE SPRAINS

(A stretch, tear, or complete rupture of one or more of the ligaments that hold the bones of the ankle joint together)

If you twist your ankle and experience a sudden sharp pain followed by swelling, you may have sustained an ankle sprain.

The most common type of ankle sprain is the inversion sprain—when someone rolls over on the outside of his or her ankle. As with all sprains, ankle sprains are classified according to severity—first, second, or third degree.

Symptoms:

- First-degree ankle sprain—Mild pain and disability, tenderness, and localized swelling. There is no instability in the ankle, no bruising, and little loss of function.
- Second-degree ankle sprain—A tearing sensation, pop, or snap is felt as the athlete rolls over on his or her ankle. There is swelling over the ankle and tenderness. Bruising begins three to four days after the injury occurs. There is some difficulty walking on the ankle.
- Third-degree ankle sprain—In many cases, the joint subluxates (slips out of place and then slips back in). There is swelling over the entire outer aspect of the ankle joint, severe tenderness, and instability. It will be extremely difficult to walk using the ankle.

Concerns:

- Unless treated properly, sprained ankles can become chronically unstable, leading to recurrent sprains.
- The same mechanism that can cause a sprain may also cause a fracture. Any sprain with severe swelling and pain needs to be x-rayed to rule out a fracture.
- An inversion sprain can tear the peroneal retinaculum, the band of tissue that holds the peroneal tendons in place, which may lead to recurrent peroneal tendon subluxations (see pages 121-124).

Treatment:

What you can do

- RICE is the cornerstone of treatment for sprains.
- If the sprain is mild, start rehabilitation exercises within 24 to 48 hours.
- If the sprain is either second or third degree (see "Symptoms"), seek medical attention.
- For relief of minor to moderate pain, take acetaminophen or ibuprofen as label-directed, or for the relief of pain *and* inflammation, take aspirin if tolerated.
- After returning to sports, wear a brace.

What the doctor can do

- The doctor should x-ray the joint to rule out a fracture.
- Once a fracture is ruled out, the doctor should start the athlete on a rehabilitation program as soon as pain allows.
- The doctor should also recommend a removable splint to prevent reinjury of the ankle. The runner should wear the splint for six weeks after the injury.

Rehabilitation:

- As soon as pain allows, engage in cardiovascular exercise that does not involve twisting and turning motions or the risk of respraining the ankle, and, making allowances for the injured area, continue as usual with strength and flexibility conditioning.
- Exercises to rehabilitate an ankle sprain should focus on stretching the muscles and tendons in the calf and heel cord area in back of the lower leg (gastro-soleus/Achilles tendon unit), which facilitate upward bending, or dorsiflexion, of the ankle. To prevent ankle sprains, it is important to be able to dorsiflex the ankle at least 15 degrees above a right angle. It is also important to strengthen the muscles that resist the ankle being turned outward, the peroneal muscles (peroneal longus, peroneal brevis), which are located on the outer side of the lower leg. These can be strengthened using rubber tubing (see pages 44-45).
- After a first-degree sprain, start rehabilitation exercises within 24 hours of the injury.
- After a second-degree sprain, start rehabilitation exercises within 24 to 48 hours.
- After a third-degree sprain in which the ligament has totally ruptured, start rehabilitation exercises one to three weeks after the

injury. Along with the exercises described, use a stationary bicycle, inversion or eversion training, and a wobble-board.

Recovery time:

- First-degree sprain: Four to six weeks.
- Second-degree sprain: Four to eight weeks.
- Third-degree sprain: Six to twelve weeks.

Taping Versus Bracing

Preventing a runner from respraining his or her ankle was once done by taping it before running. This was inconvenient, especially for recreational athletes without the benefit of an athletic trainer to tape the ankle. During the last decade or so, more convenient alternatives to taping have emerged, most notably the pneumatic air brace made by Aircast.

There are several disadvantages with taping that support the use of prefabricated braces:

- Adhesive taping loses up to 50 percent of its original support after 10 minutes of exercise.
- Taping cannot be done by the athletes themselves; it requires the assistance of a skilled "taper."
- In the long run, it is more expensive to tape every time before exercise than to purchase a prefabricated brace (taping also requires underwrap or skin lubricant, heel or lace pads, and scissors to remove the tape).
- Taping is more more time consuming than strapping on a brace.
- Studies have shown that braces are more effective in providing support for the ankle. Braces are equally effective as or better than tape in preventing resprained ankles and provide self-confidence to athletes with "bad ankles."

Overuse Ankle Injuries

Overuse ankle injuries now rival acute ankle injuries for the attention of doctors. Rarely seen by doctors until the fitness boom, overuse ankle injuries are caused by the repetitive motions involved in many of the sports that have grown in popularity, especially running.

Overuse ankle injuries are primarily tendinitis conditions of the long tendons that cross the ankle joint from the strong muscles in the lower leg.

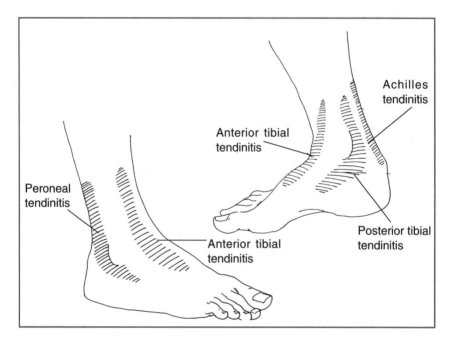

Overuse ankle injuries are usually caused by an intensive running schedule, but can be caused by intrinsic risk factors such as poor conditioning or muscle imbalances around the ankle and anatomical abnormalities in the foot area such as flat feet, feet that roll inward when the athlete runs, or high arches. All these conditions can place excessive stress on the tendons in the ankle area.

Tight posterior tibialis muscles can cause posterior tibial tendinitis, an inflammation of the tendon that runs down the back of the larger lower leg bone (the tibia) from the tibialis posterior muscle to the inner side of the foot. Similarly, tight peroneal muscles can lead to peroneal tendinitis, an inflammation of the tendon that runs behind the outer ankle bone.

As with overuse foot injuries, atypical arches are among the most common anatomical abnormalities that can cause overuse injuries in the ankle area. The runner with flat feet or feet that excessively roll inward (pronate) when they run is at greater risk of sustaining posterior tibial tendinitis because of the stress such a gait places on the posterior tibial tendon on the inner side of the foot. Conversely, bow legs or high arches that cause the feet to roll outward (supinate) when running puts the person at greater risk of sustaining peroneal tendinitis because of the stress such a gait places on the peroneal tendon on the outer side of the ankle.

The extrinsic risk factors usually associated with overuse ankle injuries are training errors, inappropriate workout structure, and improper footwear. (For a general discussion of intrinsic and extrinsic risk factors involved in overuse running injuries, see chapter 1; injury prevention guidelines can be found in chapter 2.)

POSTERIOR TIBIAL TENDINITIS

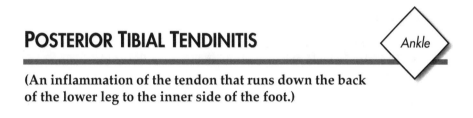

(An inflammation of the tendon that runs down the back of the lower leg to the inner side of the foot.)

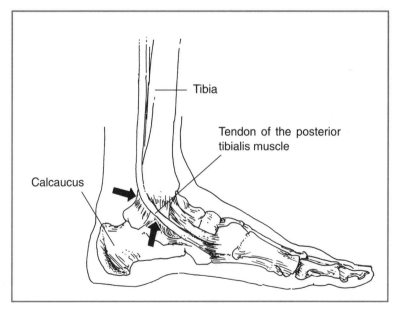

If you have pain, a creaking sensation (crepitus), and tenderness where the tendon attaches to the navicular bone or behind the inner ankle bone, you may have posterior tibial tendinitis.

This condition is usually precipitated by an intensive training schedule, although it is more likely to occur if one or more of the following risk factors are present:

INTRINSIC   Anatomical abnormalities—Flat feet, hypermobile feet.

Poor conditioning or muscle imbalances—Tight posterior tibialis muscles.

EXTRINSIC   Training error—Excessive increase in the frequency, intensity, or duration of training, including the hardness of the running surface.

Improper footwear—Worn-out shoes.

Symptoms:

- Onset of symptoms is gradual.
- The runner feels pain over the inner side of the ankle during running.
- The runner feels tenderness over the point where the tendon attaches to the navicular bone on the inside of the foot, as well as where the tendon passes behind the ankle bone.
- As the condition worsens, a creaking sensation (crepitus) develops in the area.

Concerns:

- Athletes often confuse this condition with shin splints. Unless it is recognized for what it is and treated accordingly, it can become extremely troublesome to overcome.

Treatment:

What you can do

- Suspend running schedule for two weeks, but do not completely discontinue exercise (see "Rehabilitation").
- Ice massage the area for 48 to 72 hours; then apply moist heat.
- For relief of minor to moderate pain, take acetaminophen or ibuprofen as label-directed, or for the relief of pain *and* inflammation, take aspirin if tolerated.
- For flat feet that may be causing the condition, obtain semirigid shoe inserts (orthotics) that support the arch and decrease the tendency to run on the inside of the feet.
- When all symptoms are gone, gradually return to running.

What the doctor can do

- Depending on the nature and severity of the condition, the doctor may recommend or prescribe RICE, anti-inflammatories, or immobilization of the ankle in a cast for two to three weeks.
- If the tendon sheath is constricted, surgery may be performed to make the tendon glide more smoothly inside it. After surgery, the ankle is immobilized for five to ten days, at which time rehabilitation begins.

Rehabilitation:

- Engage in cardiovascular exercise that does not aggravate the condition, and, making allowances for the injured area, continue as usual with strength and flexibility conditioning.
- Engage in a flexibility program for the entire lower extremities. If pain persists for more than two weeks, consult a certified sports doctor (see pages 83-86). The doctor will prescribe an exercise program to alleviate muscle imbalances or strength and flexibility deficits that may be the underlying causes of the condition. The rehabilitation exercises may be supervised by a physical therapist or done independently. Particular attention should be paid to stretching the muscles and tendons in the calf and heel cord area in back of the lower leg (gastro-soleus/Achilles tendon unit). It is also important to strengthen the peroneal muscles (peroneal longus, peroneal brevis), which are located on the outer side of the lower leg. These can be strengthened using rubber tubing (see pages 44-45). Stretching and strengthening the posterior tibialis muscle itself is also important.

Recovery time:

- In the cases of mild to moderate tendinitis, the condition can take anywhere from 4 to 6 weeks to clear up.
- After surgery, the athlete can go back to sports within 12 to 14 weeks.

PERONEAL TENDON SUBLUXATION

Ankle

(A process in which the tendon slips in and out of the groove created by the peroneal retinaculum behind the outer ankle bone.)

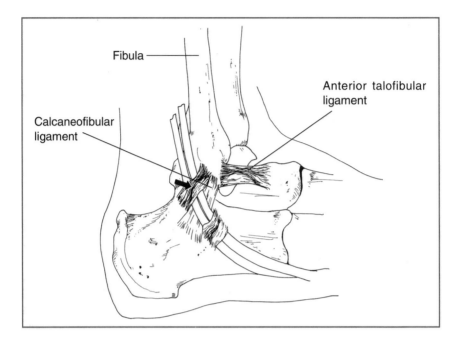

Fibula

Anterior talofibular
ligament

Calcaneofibular
ligament

If you have pain behind your outer ankle bone when you run, pain that becomes especially acute when you feel the peroneal tendon slipping out of its groove and over the ankle bone, you may be experiencing peroneal tendon subluxation.

An ankle sprain that did not fully heal may cause this condition. When the sprain took place, the peroneal retinaculum—the band of tissue that holds the tendons in place—may have torn.

This condition may also be caused if the runner performs other activities that stretch the tendons on the outside of the ankle out of shape. For instance, spending excessive time balancing on the outer edges of the feet can stretch the tendons. The subluxations occur more and more often as the peroneal tendons are stretched out of shape and slip back and forth over the ankle joint.

A naturally shallow groove behind the outer ankle bone may also cause this condition.

If the tendon does not return to its natural position, this is an acute dislocation. See a doctor. Do not try to put the tendon back in place!

Symptoms:

- Pain is felt behind the ankle bone when turning the foot upward and downward.

- The pain is especially acute when the tendon slips forward out of its groove and over the ankle bone.
- The athlete can often make this happen by simultaneously turning the foot outward and bending it upward, or by pressing the tendons from behind with the thumb.
- There should be no instability in the joint (this would signify a sprain).
- There may be direct pain when pressing on the tendon.

Concerns:

- The more often this injury occurs, the more the tendons get stretched, leading to a cycle of reoccurrence.

Treatment:

What you can do

- Seek medical attention, as surgery is usually required to correct this condition.

What the doctor can do

- Surgery is usually required to correct a subluxing peroneal tendon. When the patient has a naturally narrow groove behind the ankle bone, the surgeon deepens it by rasping out part of the tissue behind the ankle bone. Alternatively, the surgeon may decide to make the ankle bone larger by cutting out a portion of the bone and repositioning it so it juts out farther.
- After surgery, the athlete is put in a removable splint for six weeks so he or she can start rehabilitation exercises after three weeks.

Rehabilitation:

- Three weeks after surgery, the athlete can begin gentle range of motion and strengthening exercises. The focus should be on stretching the peroneal muscles on the outer side of the lower leg, as well as the muscles and tendons in the calf and heel cord area in back of the lower leg (gastro-soleus/Achilles tendon unit). Also, the athlete can strengthen the muscles that turn the foot upward and inward at the ankle bone, primarily the anterior tibialis, the one that runs up and down the front of the lower leg just to the outside of the shinbone.

Recovery time:

- The athlete can usually return to sports 12 to 16 weeks after surgery.

PERONEAL TENDINITIS
Ankle

(An inflammation of the tendon that runs behind the outer ankle bone.)

If you have pain, tenderness, and a creaking sensation behind the outer ankle bone when running (the pain may radiate up the outer side of the lower leg), you may have peroneal tendinitis.

An intensive training schedule usually causes this condition, though it is more likely to occur if one or more of the following risk factors exist:

INTRINSIC   Anatomical abnormalities—Bow legs or high arches (both make the athlete run on the outside of the feet, thus stressing the peroneal tendons).

Poor conditioning or muscle imbalances—Tight peroneal tendons.

EXTRINSIC   Training errors - Excessive increases in the frequency, intensity, or duration of the running regimen, including the hardness of the running surface.

Improper footwear—Worn-out shoes or shoes that rub against the peroneal tendons.

Symptoms:

- Onset of symptoms is gradual.
- Pain and tenderness occur behind the outer ankle when running. This pain may radiate up the outer side of the lower leg.
- As the condition worsens, a creaking sensation (crepitus) develops in the area.

Concerns:

- Unless treated early, this condition can deteriorate to the point where surgery becomes necessary.

Treatment:

What you can do

- Suspend running schedule for two weeks, but do not completely discontinue exercise (see "Rehabilitation").
- Continue cardiovascular exercise that does not aggravate the tendinitis.
- Ice the tendinitis for 48 to 72 hours; then apply moist heat.
- For relief of minor to moderate pain, take acetaminophen or ibuprofen as label-directed, or for the relief of pain *and* inflammation, take aspirin if tolerated.
- For high arches that may be causing the condition, obtain shoe inserts (orthotics) that support the arch and decrease the tendency to run on the outside of the feet.
- When all symptoms are gone, gradually return to running.

What the doctor can do

- To correct the initial stages of pain and inflammation, the doctor should prescribe RICE, followed by a conditioning program to develop strength and flexibility in the muscles.

Rehabilitation:

- Engage in cardiovascular exercise that does not aggravate the condition, such as swimming, and, making allowances for the injured area, continue as usual with strength and flexibility conditioning.
- Engage in a flexibility program for the entire lower extremities. If pain persists for more than two weeks, consult a certified sports doctor (see pages 83-86). The doctor will prescribe an exercise program to alleviate muscle imbalances or strength and flexibility deficits that may be the underlying causes of the condition. The rehabilitation exercises may be supervised by a physical therapist or done independently. Concentrate on stretching the peroneal muscles on the outer side of the lower leg, as well as the muscles and tendons in the calf and heel cord area in back of the lower leg (gastro-soleus/Achilles tendon unit). Also, strengthen the muscles that turn the foot upward and inward at the ankle bone, primarily the anterior tibialis, which runs up and down the front of the lower leg just to the outside of the shinbone.

Recovery time:

With the appropriate treatment, this condition should clear up within four to six weeks.

Ankle

OSTEOCHONDRITIS DISSECANS OF THE ANKLE

(Damage to the joint surface, which if allowed to worsen may lead to chips of bone and cartilage falling into the joint.)

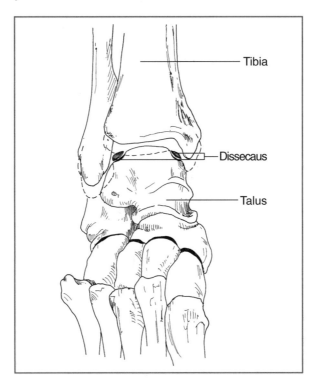

If over the course of several months you develop pain and swelling in the ankle joint when you run, and the symptoms intensify after you stop running, you may have osteochondritis dissecans.

This condition is caused by the ends of the bones in the joint bumping together. This can create a small crater in the large ankle bone (talus) with pieces of bone and cartilage around it—rather like a divot in the ground caused by a missed golf stroke. Osteochondritis refers to the damage caused by the friction, while dissecans are the loose pieces around the crater. If the stress continues, a dissecans composed of bone and cartilage may break off and fall into the joint.

In adults, bumping together of the ends of the bones may cause divots, though it is rare that pieces of bone and cartilage dislodge and fall into the joint. But in children, whose joint surfaces are much softer because they are made up of growing bone that has not yet hardened, there is a much greater chance that a portion of bone and cartilage can dislodge and fall into the joint. Children between the ages of 12 and 16 are especially at risk because of the relative softness of the ends of their bones.

Symptoms:

- Onset of symptoms is gradual, usually taking place over a period of three to six months.
- Pain and swelling are felt during exercise and may intensify afterward. The ankle may often stiffen after sports activity.
- There is no instability or loss of range of motion.
- If the fragment has detached, the joint may occasionally lock.

Concerns:

- Ignoring this condition will allow a simple divot to deteriorate to the point where pieces of bone and cartilage break off and fall into the joint, a condition that almost always requires surgery if the athlete wants to continue in sports.

Treatment:

What you can do

- Suspend running schedule or any activity that aggravates the ankle, but do not completely discontinue exercise (see "Rehabilitation").
- For relief of minor to moderate pain, take acetaminophen or ibuprofen as label-directed, or for the relief of pain *and* inflammation, take aspirin if tolerated.
- Seek medical attention.

What the doctor can do

- The doctor should confirm the diagnosis with an X ray, CAT scan, MRI, or bone scan.
- If no fragments have detached, the doctor may immobilize the ankle for four to eight weeks to allow the damage to repair itself.
- If the symptoms continue for more than six months, surgery may be considered.

Surgical options

The surgeon performs either an open procedure or arthroscopy to remove the fragment. If the fragment is small, simple removal is sufficient, after which the surgeon drills tiny holes in the crater to stimulate regrowth of the bone cartilage. If the fragment is larger than half an inch across, it will be necessary to pin it back in place to ensure that the joint works properly.

If only drilling is done, the ankle is immobilized for four to six weeks. When a fragment is pinned in place, the athlete should avoid weightbearing activity for at least six weeks.

Rehabilitation:

- Maintain all-around strength in the muscles around the ankle through nonweightbearing cardiovascular activity and stretching and strengthening exercises that do not excessively stress the joint.
- If the condition is handled nonsurgically, rehabilitation exercises can start as soon as pain abates.
- After surgery to remove loose fragments or drill holes in the crater, the runner can begin rehabilitation exercises five to seven days later under the supervision of a physical therapist. If a large fragment is pinned in place, exercises supervised by a physical therapist should begin in three weeks.

Recovery time:

- Nonoperative recovery time: 6 weeks or more.
- After surgical removal of fragments or drilling: 8 to 12 weeks.
- After fixation of a large fragment: 8 to 12 weeks.

6

Lower Leg Injuries

Overuse injuries of the lower leg commonly seen in runners include tendinitis of the Achilles tendon, as well as a variety of disorders traditionally lumped together under the heading shin splints.

The term shin splints has traditionally been used to describe any chronic, exercise-related lower leg pain. This umbrella diagnosis may encompass several quite different conditions, including inflammation of the tissue that covers the shinbone, stress fractures of either bone of the lower leg, and compartment syndromes that may affect any of the four muscle compartments in the lower leg. Although athletes still use the term shin splints, sports doctors no longer use it because it is too vague. Doctors now place lower leg pain in four categories—medial tibial (inner shinbone) pain syndrome, compartment syndromes, stress fractures, and tendinitis. Runners may feel the symptoms of these conditions in the inner side, outer side, front, or back of the lower leg.

Pain in the inner side of the leg is generally caused by inflammations of the tissue that covers the tibia (periostitis), inflammation of the tibial posterior muscle-tendon, stress fractures of the tibia or fibula, or posterior compartment syndrome.

Pain at the front of the lower leg is usually anterior compartment syndrome or stress fracture. Pain at the outer side of the lower leg is usually lateral compartment syndrome, stress fracture, or tendinitis.

Pain behind the leg is usually posterior superficial compartment syndrome.

Each condition—tendinitis, periostitis, stress fracture, and compartment syndrome—has different symptoms, causes, diagnosis, treatment, and rehabilitation.

129

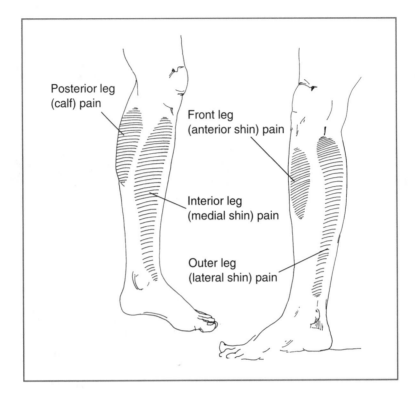

Posterior leg
(calf) pain

Front leg
(anterior shin) pain

Interior leg
(medial shin) pain

Outer leg
(lateral shin) pain

An intensive running schedule usually causes overuse injuries in the lower leg, but intrinsic risk factors such as poor conditioning or muscle imbalances and anatomical abnormalities may be the cause. Tight Achilles tendons are a primary cause of Achilles tendinitis, one of the most common running injuries. Inflexibility can also exist in lesser-known soft tissue groups, such as the fascial walls of the muscle compartments and the periosteum of the tibia, which can cause compartment syndrome and periostitis, respectively.

Significantly, running itself may cause tightness and imbalances in certain muscle groups, especially those in front of the hip (psoas muscles), in back of the thigh (hamstrings), and in back of the lower leg (calves/ Achilles tendon unit). Such tightness may cause a person to run in a way that may cause injuries. Specifically, he or she may have a much briefer-than-normal foot strike, which causes the foot to absorb excessive stress with each step. The feet may absorb this stress, which may cause problems in that area, or the stress may be transmitted to other parts of the lower extremities, including the lower leg. As a result of these transmitted stresses, stress fractures may occur in one or both of the lower leg bones.

Stress Fractures in Runners

These are the most common stress fractures seen in runners, based on two doctors experiences with 1,000 runners:

Tibia (front shinbone)		34%
Upper tibia	7%	
Upper-mid tibia	12%	
Mid tibia	4%	
Lower tibia	11%	
Fibula (rear shinbone)		24%
Metatarsals (foot/toe)		18%
Second	7%	
Third	11%	
Pelvis		6%
Others		
Fourth or fifth metatarsals		4%
Pars, sesamoid, navicular, talus		___
		86%

Courtesy of Drs. M.E. Blazine, R.S. Watanbe, A.M. McBryde Jr.

Anatomical abnormalities such as flat feet are often responsible for overuse running injuries in the lower leg. People whose feet excessively turn inward (pronate) when they run—characteristic of people with flat feet—are more likely to develop pain in the front of the lower leg because of the contortions the lower leg has to perform to carry them in a straight line.

Bowed lower leg bones, known as tibia vara, may also increase the chance of a runner sustaining an overuse injury in the lower legs.

Flat feet may contribute to posterior tibial tendinitis, another condition grouped under the umbrella term shin splints. Part of the role of the posterior tibial muscle is to provide the arch of the foot with support. In runners with flat feet, that muscle and its tendon must work extra hard to support the arch and prevent the heel from turning in. The pain occurs on the inner side of the lower shin. Because the runner feels the symptoms of posterior tibial tendinitis in the ankle area, this condition is covered in chapter 5.

The extrinsic risk factors associated with overuse running injuries of the lower leg include training errors, inappropriate workout structure, and improper footwear. (For a general discussion of intrinsic and extrinsic risk factors involved in overuse running injuries, see chapter 1; injury prevention guidelines can be found in chapter 2.)

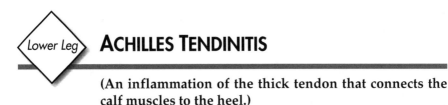

‹Lower Leg› ACHILLES TENDINITIS

(An inflammation of the thick tendon that connects the calf muscles to the heel.)

If you have a creaking sensation in your Achilles tendon in back of your lower leg, and pain, aching, and soreness before, during, and after running, and the symptoms intensify when walking uphill or climbing stairs, you may have Achilles tendinitis.

The repetitive stretching of the tendon that occurs in running causes Achilles tendinitis. The condition is especially prevalent in athletes over 30 because of degenerative changes in the tendons beginning between the ages of 25 and 30, which make them tighter and weaker.

An intensive running schedule usually precipitates Achilles tendinitis, though it is more likely to occur if one or more of the following risk factors exist:

INTRINSIC   Anatomical abnormalities—Flat feet, high arches.

Poor conditioning or muscle imbalances—Tight, weak calf muscles or Achilles tendons.

EXTRINSIC   Training errors—Rapid increases in frequency, intensity, or duration of training, including changing to a harder running surface or a banked running surface.

Inappropriate workout structure—Not stretching out the calf muscles or Achilles tendons before running.

Improper footwear—Worn-out running shoes.

Symptoms:

- Onset of symptoms is gradual.
- Pain occurs with use, and there may be swelling over the tendon.
- As the condition worsens, there may be redness over the tendon.
- There may be a creaking sensation in the tendon, which can be felt with the fingers when the ankle is bent backward and forward.
- If the athlete ignores the condition, the following symptoms may develop: (1) pain, aching, and stiffness before, during, and after exercise; (2) the tendon may become tender to the touch; and (3) the pain intensifies when walking uphill or climbing stairs.

Concerns:

Unless caught early, this condition is extremely difficult to overcome.

Treatment:

What you can do

- For the first 48 to 72 hours, suspend running schedule and administer 20-minute ice massage sessions. However, do not completely discontinue exercise (see "Rehabilitation").
- After 72 hours, begin moist heat treatments and use a neoprene heat retainer.
- For relief of minor to moderate pain, take acetaminophen or ibuprofen as label-directed, or for the relief of pain *and* inflammation, take aspirin if tolerated.
- Seven to ten days after the initial symptoms, begin the stretching and strengthening program outlined in chapter 2.
- Wear shoes with a half-inch heel wedge to relieve tension on the tendon (wear the lifts in both shoes to avoid problems arising from unequal leg lengths).
- Continue cardiovascular activities that do not stress the Achilles tendon, such as swimming and cycling.
- After going back to running, stretch before exercise and ice the tendon afterward if there is pain.
- If the condition does not clear up within two weeks, consult a sports doctor.

What the doctor can do

- If there is any question about the diagnosis, the doctor should order an MRI.

- If the above treatment regimen does not work, the doctor may, depending on the underlying cause of the condition, prescribe
  —anti-inflammatories,
  —orthotics (store-bought leather longitudinal arch supports are often all the runner needs; runners with more severe or complex foot abnormalities may need custom-made rigid orthotics), or
  —physical therapy (if the patient has tight or weak calf muscles or Achilles tendons).
- The doctor may also recommend heel wedges to relieve stress on the tendon.
- If the condition is severe, the runner may be put in a cast for three to six weeks.
- If the condition persists for more than two to three months, a surgical procedure may be considered. The doctor will cut open the end of the tendon's sheath to give it more room and trim the inflamed tissue from the tendon.

Cortisone injections are not recommended for Achilles tendinitis since they may weaken the tendon and cause it to rupture.

Rehabilitation:

- Engage in cardiovascular exercise that does not aggravate the condition, such as swimming or cycling, and, making allowances for the injured area, continue as usual with strength and flexibility conditioning.
- Engage in a flexibility program for the entire lower extremities. If pain persists for more than two weeks, consult a certified sports doctor (see pages 83-86). The doctor should prescribe an exercise program to alleviate muscle imbalances or strength and flexibility deficits that may be the underlying causes of the condition. The rehabilitation exercises may be supervised by a physical therapist or done independently. Particular attention should be paid to stretching the Achilles tendons and strengthening the muscles in the lower leg that bend the foot upward at the ankle, especially the anterior tibialis.

Recovery time:

If caught early and if the cause of the condition is addressed, Achilles tendinitis can clear up within one to two weeks. However, chronic conditions may take up to six months to overcome and often will never clear up unless surgery is performed.

MEDIAL TIBIAL PAIN SYNDROME (PERIOSTITIS OF THE SHINBONE)

Lower Leg

(An inflammation of the membrane [periosteum] that covers the shinbone [tibia].)

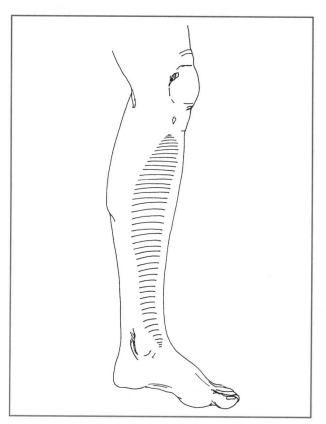

If you have pain, tenderness, and possibly swelling on the inner side of the shin, especially pronounced over the bottom half of the lower leg, you may have medial tibial pain syndrome, sometimes known as periostitis of the shinbone.

This condition was once referred to as shin splints, though this term is misleading because it covered a variety of ailments in the lower leg. Pain in this area is now more properly referred to as medial tibial pain syndrome, which means pain in the inside front of the lower leg.

The repetitive pounding of the feet on the running surface, transmitting force to the shinbone, causes medial tibial pain syndrome.

An intensive running schedule may precipitate medial tibial pain syndrome, though it is more likely to occur if one or more of the following risk factors exist:

INTRINSIC   Anatomical abnormalities—Flat feet, high arches.

Incorrect running technique—Running on the toes or using a shorter-than-usual foot strike.

EXTRINSIC   Training error—Excessively increasing the frequency, intensity, or duration of the training regimen, especially changing from a softer to a harder running surface (such as grass to pavement).

Improper footwear—Worn-out shoes, or shoes inappropriate for foot type.

Symptoms:

- Onset of symptoms is gradual.
- The runner experiences pain, tenderness, and possibly swelling on the inner side of the shin, especially pronounced over the bottom half of the lower leg.
- Pain can be triggered when the toes or ankle are bent downward against resistance.
- Pain abates when the athlete is at rest, but returns with running and jumping activities. When allowed to deteriorate, the runner eventually feels the condition before, during, and after activity.

Concerns:

- Allowed to deteriorate, this condition can become chronic and thus difficult to clear up.

Treatment:

What you can do

- Suspend running schedule, but do not discontinue exercise entirely (see "Rehabilitation").
- For the first 48 to 72 hours, administer ice massage.
- For relief of minor to moderate pain, take acetaminophen or ibuprofen as label-directed, or for the relief of pain *and* inflammation, take aspirin if tolerated.
- Refrain from running until there is absolutely no pain on the inner side of the lower leg when running and no tenderness to the touch.

- When you resume running, do so on a soft surface (ideally grass) and cut the frequency, intensity, and duration of the training regimen by half, building back to the original training regimen over six weeks.
- If the symptoms persist for two weeks despite the above measures, consult a sports doctor.

What the doctor can do

- The doctor should first rule out other possible causes of lower leg pain, notably stress fractures and compartment syndrome.
- Once medial tibial pain syndrome has been confirmed, the doctor may recommend or prescribe

    —ice massage and then heat treatments with a physical therapist,
    —a two-week course of anti-inflammatories,
    —orthotics (store-bought leather longitudinal arch supports are often all the runner needs; runners with more severe or complex foot abnormalities may need custom-made rigid orthotics),
    —a more appropriate shoe,
    —physical therapy (if the runner has strength or flexibility deficits, or tight or weak muscles), or
    —a cortisone injection under the periosteum.

- If none of the above measures are successful, the doctor may perform surgery to separate the periosteum from the inner side of the shinbone.

Rehabilitation:

- Engage in nonweightbearing cardiovascular activities such as swimming or stationary biking (when cycling, the foot should be positioned so the _heel_ is over the pedal, not the forefoot), and, making allowances for the injured area, continue as usual with strength and flexibility conditioning.
- Engage in a flexibility program for the entire lower extremities. If pain persists for more than two weeks, consult a certified sports doctor (see pages 83-86). The doctor should prescribe an exercise program to alleviate muscle imbalances or strength and flexibility deficits that may be the underlying causes of the condition. The rehabilitation exercises may be supervised by a physical therapist or done independently. Particular attention should be paid to stretching the heel cords (Achilles tendons) in back of the lower leg, and strengthening the muscles that turn the foot upward and

inward at the ankle bone, primarily the anterior tibialis, the one that runs up and down the front of the lower leg just to the outside of the shinbone.

Recovery time:

If caught early, the condition will clear up within one to two weeks. However, chronic conditions may take as long as six months to resolve and sometimes will never clear up unless surgery is performed.

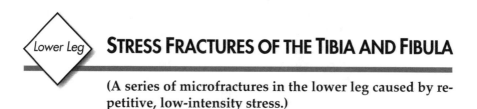

STRESS FRACTURES OF THE TIBIA AND FIBULA

(A series of microfractures in the lower leg caused by repetitive, low-intensity stress.)

If you have pain and highly localized tenderness in the top third of the shinbone, you may have a stress fracture of the tibia; if you feel the same symptoms on the outside of the lower leg, just above the ankle, you may have a stress fracture of the fibula.

When the stress fracture takes place in the tibia (the larger of the two lower leg bones), it occurs in the top two-thirds of that bone. In the fibula (the smaller of the two bones), stress fractures usually take place two or three inches above the lateral malleolus (the outer ankle bone). Page 88 describes two possible theories to explain how stress fractures develop.

An intensive running schedule usually precipitates stress fractures in the lower leg, though they are more likely to occur if one or more of the following risk factors exist:

INTRINSIC   Anatomical abnormalities—Flat feet, high arches, or leg length inequalities.

Poor conditioning or muscle imbalances—Tight calf muscles and Achilles tendons; overly strong and tight muscles in front of the hip (psoas), in back of the thigh (hamstrings), and in the calf and heel cord area in back of the lower leg (gastro-soleus/Achilles tendon unit), which can interfere with running technique and transmit excessive stress to the lower leg.

Nutritional abuse—Women who menstruate irregularly because of poor diet and excessive exercise often develop bone thinning and are therefore at increased risk of stress fractures.

Incorrect running technique—A shorter-than-optimal foot strike that transmits excessive stress from the foot to the lower leg.

EXTRINSIC   Training errors—Excessively increasing the frequency, intensity, or duration of training regimen, especially changing from a softer to a harder running surface (such as grass to pavement).

Improper footwear—Worn-out shoes, or shoes inappropriate for foot type.

Symptoms:

- Onset of symptoms is gradual, though they may occasionally develop after a sudden increase in the intensity, frequency, or duration of an athlete's training regimen.
- When the stress fracture is in the tibia, the runner usually feels pain and highly localized tenderness at the top third of the front of the leg. When the stress fracture is in the fibula, the runner feels the same symptoms just above the ankle bone on the outside of the leg.
- Pain is especially intense during running and abates at rest.
- It may be difficult to differentiate the pain from soft tissue pain such as that of a tibial periostitis (see pages 135-138). There are two ways to tell if the pain is caused by a stress fracture. First, firmly tap the tibia or fibula above the point of tenderness: the vibration in the bone will travel to the fracture itself and be felt only at that point (in a soft tissue injury, the pain is more spread out). Second, have someone tap the underside of the heel of the affected leg: again, the vibration will travel to the stress fracture site.

Girls and women with eating disorders and menstrual irregularities are at greater risk of sustaining stress fractures (see page 191).

Concerns:

If allowed to deteriorate, stress fractures can lead to complete fractures.

Treatment:

What you can do

- Suspend running schedule, but do not discontinue exercise entirely (see "Rehabilitation").
- Administer ice massage according to the RICE prescription.
- For relief of minor to moderate pain, take acetaminophen or ibuprofen as label-directed, or for the relief of pain *and* inflammation, take aspirin if tolerated.
- If the symptoms described above are present, or if pain lasts for longer than two weeks despite ice massage, consult a sports doctor.

What the doctor can do

- The doctor should confirm the diagnosis with X rays or a bone scan. Bone scans are more effective than X rays in detecting stress fractures, because the visible changes that take place on the surface of the bone are not visible on X rays until several weeks after the actual damage occurs (in medical parlance, they are occult).
- If the diagnosis is confirmed, the doctor may recommend six weeks' rest from running, but should encourage nonweightbearing cardiovascular activities such as swimming and stationary biking.
- Depending on the underlying cause of the stress fracture, the doctor may prescribe

    —orthotics (if the cause is anatomical abnormalities),
    —physical therapy (if the cause is weak or tight muscles, or imbalances in muscle strength or flexibility), or
    —nutritional counseling (if the patient is a female who is experiencing menstrual irregularities due to an eating disorder).

- After six weeks, with at least two weeks being pain free, the doctor can recommend a return to running.

Rehabilitation:

- Engage in cardiovascular exercise that does not aggravate the condition, such as swimming, and, making allowances for the injured area, continue as usual with strength and flexibility conditioning.
- Engage in a flexibility program for the entire lower extremities. If pain persists for more than two weeks, consult a certified sports doctor (see pages 83-86). The doctor should prescribe an exercise program to alleviate muscle imbalances or strength and flexibility deficits that may be the underlying causes of the condition. The rehabilitation exercises may be supervised by a physical therapist

or done independently. Particular attention should be paid to stretching the muscles in the front of the hip (psoas), in back of the thigh (hamstrings), and the calf and heel cord area in back of the lower leg (gastro-soleus/Achilles tendon unit), which, if tight, may interfere with foot strike and transmit excessive stress from the foot to the lower leg, perhaps causing stress fractures.

Recovery time:

Stress fractures in the lower leg will take three weeks or longer to heal, although the runner should not return to running for at least six weeks, including two pain-free weeks.

COMPARTMENT SYNDROMES

⟨Lower Leg⟩

(An overswelling of the muscles in their membranous encasements, an effect that compresses the muscles and nerves within these compartments, causing tightness, numbness, and muscle weakness.)

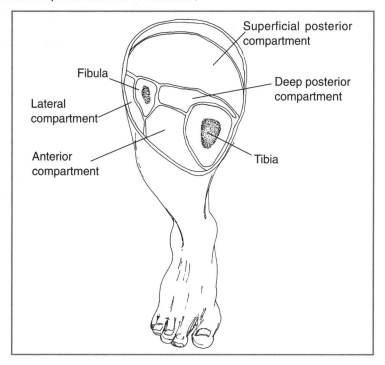

If you have an ache, sharp pain, or pressure in the front of the lower leg when running that completely abates shortly after you stop, you may have anterior compartment syndrome.

Compartment syndromes in the lower leg occur because of intensive training, which makes certain of these lower leg muscles too large for their compartments. At rest, there is no problem, but when the person with this condition runs, the muscles swell with blood. This causes pressure inside the compartments, which compresses the muscles and nerves within the compartment, and produces the characteristic symptoms of compartment syndrome. This condition can occur in any of the four compartments in the lower leg, although it is most often seen in the anterior compartment (when pain is felt on the inner side of the lower leg, the problem may lie with the posterior compartment; when it is felt on the outer side of the lower leg, the lateral compartment may be causing the condition; pain in the back of the lower leg may signify a compartment syndrome affecting the superficial posterior compartment).

An intensive running schedule usually causes compartment syndromes in the lower leg, though they are more likely to occur if one or more of the following risk factors exist:

INTRINSIC   Poor conditioning or muscle imbalances—Tight muscles in the front of the hip, back of the thigh, and back of the lower leg, which can shorten foot strike. This in turn can transmit excessive stresses to the lower leg.

Anatomical abnormalities—Naturally tight compartment walls.

EXTRINSIC   Training errors—Excessively increasing the frequency, intensity, or duration of the training regimen, especially changing from a softer to a harder running surface (such as grass to pavement).

Improper footwear—Worn-out shoes, or shoes inappropriate for foot type.

Symptoms:

- Onset of symptoms is gradual, though occasional symptoms may be extremely intense.
- The person experiences an ache, sharp pain, or pressure in the front of the lower leg when running. The symptoms completely abate when not running.

- When the condition deteriorates, there may be weakness when trying to bend the foot and toes upward and when the foot and toes are bent downward using the hands. The runner may experience numbness in the top of the foot and between the big toe and the second toe. It will become impossible to exercise for extended periods.

Concerns:

- Unless measures are taken early to manage this condition, it can deteriorate to the point where surgery is necessary if the person hopes to continue running. In severe cases of overuse compartment syndromes, the muscles can exert so much pressure on the nerves in the compartment that permanent nerve damage may occur.

Treatment:

What you can do

- Suspend running schedule and administer ice massage according to the RICE prescription. Do not completely discontinue exercise (see "Rehabilitation").
- Modify running regimen, paying particular attention to the running surface, footwear, and running technique.
- For relief of minor to moderate pain, take acetaminophen or ibuprofen as label-directed, or for the relief of pain *and* inflammation, take aspirin if tolerated.
- As soon as pain subsides, return to running. It is likely, however, that the pain will return.

What the doctor can do

- The doctor should confirm the diagnosis with a compartment syndrome test (a needle is inserted into the muscle before and after activity to measure pressure within the compartment).
- Once the diagnosis is confirmed, the doctor should advise the runner that surgery will be necessary if he or she wishes to maintain a rigorous running schedule. In this procedure, known as a fasciotomy, the doctor cuts open the compartment walls to relieve the pressure within the compartment. The procedure is done on an outpatient basis. The athlete is usually walking without crutches within a week, and may be able to return to gentle running within two weeks.

Rehabilitation:

- Engage in nonweightbearing cardiovascular exercise that does not aggravate the condition, such as swimming and stationary biking and, making allowances for the injured area, continue as usual with strength and flexibility conditioning.
- Engage in a flexibility program for the entire lower extremities. If pain persists for more than two weeks, consult a certified sports doctor (see pages 83-86). The doctor should prescribe an exercise program to alleviate muscle imbalances or strength and flexibility deficits that may be the underlying causes of the condition. The rehabilitation exercises may be supervised by a physical therapist or done independently. Particular attention should be paid to stretching the Achilles tendons.
- Start rehabilitation exercises a week after the operation.

Recovery time:

- Unless surgery is done, this condition probably will not clear up.
- After surgery, the athlete may begin gentle running after two weeks, working up to a full running schedule within four to six weeks.

Knee Injuries

The knee is the largest and most complex joint in the body. Given the enormous stresses to which it is subjected during running, it is natural that knee injuries are common among runners. The potentially debilitating consequences of a knee injury reinforce the need for a focus on prevention.

Knee overuse injuries include patellofemoral pain syndrome (kneecap pain), meniscus wear and tear, tendinitis conditions both above and below the kneecap, bursitis, and loose bodies in the knee.

Overuse knee injuries are usually caused by excessive running, but can be caused by intrinsic risk factors such as poor conditioning or muscle imbalances, and anatomical abnormalities such as a difference in leg length, abnormalities in hip rotation or the position of the kneecap, bow legs, knock knees, or flat feet.

Knee function depends on the highly complex interaction among a number of the surrounding muscles. The most important actions are performed by the quadriceps (straightening) and hamstrings (bending) in the front and back of the thigh, respectively.

Imbalances in strength or flexibility between the quadriceps or hamstrings can predispose the runner to a common overuse knee injury called patellofemoral pain syndrome, which is usually caused by the kneecap tracking improperly in its groove at the front of the bottom of the thighbone. Often, this problem is caused by the excessive tightness of the hamstring muscles in back of the thigh compared to the quadriceps muscles in front of the thigh. In such circumstances, the quadriceps cannot maintain the proper straight-ahead alignment of the lower and upper leg when the person runs; as a result, the lower leg "spins out" during the running cycle, which in turn causes excessive stress to the outer side of the kneecap.

Another common imbalance *within* the quadriceps muscle group in the front of the thigh, between the outer quadriceps muscle (vastus lateralis) and the inner quadriceps muscle (vastus medialis), can also cause kneecap problems. These two muscles run down either side of the front of the thigh and attach to the kneecap. Part of their role is to stabilize the kneecap. When one side is stronger than the other, the kneecap can be pulled to one side when the person runs. Since runners frequently have comparatively stronger, tighter outer quadriceps muscles than inner quadriceps muscles, the kneecap can be pulled to the outer side. This mechanism is a common cause of patellofemoral pain syndrome in runners.

Tightness in the iliotibial band—a thick, wide band of muscle-tendon tissue running down the outside of the thigh from the hip to just below the knee—is the underlying cause of one of the most prevalent overuse injuries of the knee in runners, a condition known as iliotibial band friction syndrome.

Anatomical abnormalities are the second most common intrinsic risk factor. Several are closely associated with overuse knee injuries in runners:

- Flat feet, or feet that excessively turn inward (pronate) when the person runs—Inward rotation of the lower leg causes the kneecap to track improperly (see page 11).
- Knock knees—Excessive inward angling at the point where the thigh and lower leg meet (Q angle) causes the runner's weight to be borne on the inside of the knee; an angle of greater than 10 degrees in men and 15 degrees in women is said to predispose that person to knee problems if he or she participates in a rigorous running regimen (see page 13).
- Bow legs—Greater distance over which the iliotibial band must stretch over the outside of the leg may cause tightness at the point where the iliotibial band crosses over the outside of the knee joint (iliotibial band friction syndrome; see page 13).
- Unequal leg length—In the longer leg, the greater distance over which the iliotibial band must stretch may cause inflammation in this tissue over the outside of the knee, perhaps causing iliotibial band friction syndrome (see pages 14-15).
- Turned-in thighbones—Inward-facing kneecaps characteristic of people with this abnormality may cause tracking problems in the kneecap (see page 12).

- Loose kneecaps, high-riding kneecaps (more often seen in very tall people), shallow femoral groove (the groove at the bottom of the thighbone in which the kneecap lies is too shallow)—All three of these anatomical abnormalities can cause the kneecap to track improperly, sometimes so severely that the kneecap completely slips in and out of its proper position (subluxation)
- "Miserable malalignment syndrome"—The combination of thighs that turn inward from the hip, knock knees, and flat feet can cause many problems.

Extrinsic risk factors associated with overuse knee injuries usually involve training errors, inappropriate workout structure, and improper footwear. (For a general discussion of intrinsic and extrinsic risk factors involved in overuse running injuries, see chapter 1; injury prevention guidelines can be found in chapter 2.)

ILIOTIBIAL BAND FRICTION SYNDROME ⟨ *Knee* ⟩

(An inflammation of the iliotibial band where it rubs against the outer part of the knee joint.)

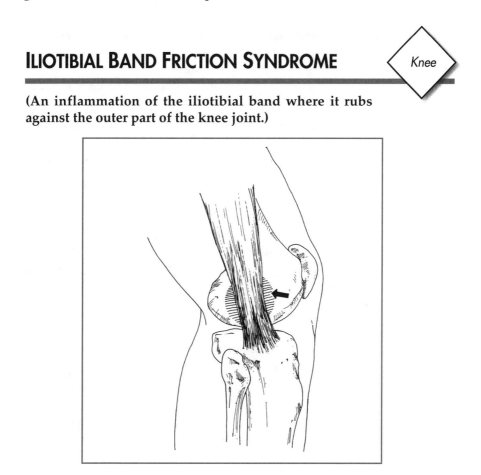

If you have a tightness on the outside of your knee that burns or stings when you run, you may have iliotibial band friction syndrome.

Iliotibial band friction syndrome is caused by the repetitive bending and straightening of the knee that occurs in running, which causes the iliotibial band to rub against the outer side of the knee.

An intensive running schedule usually causes this condition, though it is more likely to occur if one or more of the following risk factors exist:

INTRINSIC   Anatomical abnormalities—Abnormally large trochanter, unequal leg length, bow legs (both conditions increase the tightness of the iliotibial band over the outside of the knee; in the case of unequal leg length, the tightness occurs in the longer leg).

Poor conditioning or muscle imbalances—Tight iliotibial band.

EXTRINSIC   Training error—Excessively increasing the frequency, intensity, or duration of the running regimen, including running on a sloped surface (the problem will occur in the downside leg of the runner).

Inappropriate workout structure—Not stretching out the iliotibial band before running.

Improper footwear—Worn-out running shoes.

Symptoms:

- Onset of symptoms is gradual.
- The runner feels tightness on the outer side of the knee. This sensation burns or stings during running.
- Discomfort will eventually cause the person to stop running, and the symptoms will abate. Pain recurs when the person resumes running.
- The pain is especially acute when running downhill or walking down stairs.
- In its most severe form, pain from this condition will force the runner to walk with the injured leg fully straightened to relieve friction of the iliotibial band over the outer side of the knee joint.

Treatment:

What you can do

For a mild case of iliotibial band friction syndrome, do the following:

- Cease the activity that causes the condition, or reduce training to a pain-free level. Do not completely discontinue exercise (see "Rehabilitation").
- Ice the knee at least three times a day for 20 minutes at a time.
- Begin a strength and flexibility program for the iliotibial band, focusing on rehabilitation exercise, using the iliotibial stretch (see below). Do these exercises six times a day, holding each stretch for 30 seconds at a time.

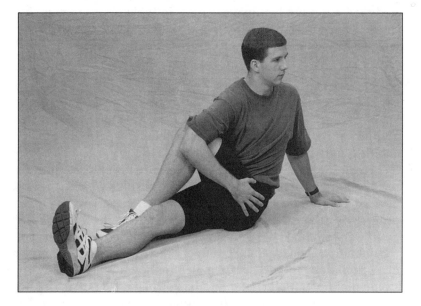

- Change running surfaces where appropriate, especially avoiding sloped surfaces.
- For relief of minor to moderate pain, take acetaminophen or ibuprofen as label-directed, or for the relief of pain *and* inflammation, take aspirin if tolerated.
- If the condition does not clear up within two weeks, the inflammation may be severe. In such cases, consult a sports doctor.

What the doctor can do

- Even when the condition is relatively severe, most sports doctors treat this condition nonsurgically. The doctor may recommend or prescribe
  —anti-inflammatories,
  —a knee immobilizer and crutches for three to five days (the knee immobilizer should be removed for icing and stretching and strengthening exercises),
  —orthotics (if the problem is caused by bow legs or unequal leg length), or
  —a cortisone injection.

Surgery is rarely required for iliotibial band friction syndrome, and then only when all other methods fail. The surgical procedure to correct this condition is an iliotibial band release, in which the surgeon cuts open the back portion of the iliotibial band, thereby reducing the tension over the knee.

Rehabilitation:

- Engage in cardiovascular activities that do not involve repetitive knee bending and straightening, such as swimming, and, making allowances for the injured area, continue as usual with strength and flexibility conditioning.
- Engage in a flexibility program for the entire lower extremities. If pain persists for more than two weeks, consult a certified sports doctor (see pages 83-86). The doctor should prescribe an exercise program to alleviate muscle imbalances or strength and flexibility deficits that may be the underlying causes of the condition. The rehabilitation exercises may be supervised by a physical therapist or done independently. Particular attention should be paid to stretching the iliotibial band and hamstrings, and strengthening the muscles in front of the thigh (quadriceps) with straight leg raises and the muscles on the outside of the hip that help raise the hip outward (tensor fascia latae, gluteus minimus, gluteus maximus).

Recovery time:

Mild cases of iliotibial band friction syndrome may clear up within three to five days of starting rest, ice, and stretching. More severe cases may take up to two weeks to resolve. Very severe cases of iliotibial band friction syndrome may take up to six months to clear up.

MENISCUS INJURIES

Knee

(Damage to one or both of the two flat, crescent-shaped pieces of cartilage that lie in the knee joint between the thighbone and large shinbone.)

If you experience pain on the inner side of the knee joint when running, and your knee sometimes clicks or locks in place momentarily, you may have a torn meniscus.

Usually a single episode of trauma, often a violent bend of the knee, causes the damage to the meniscus, which is then aggravated by repetitive twisting and turning in sports and daily activities. In many cases, the symptoms do not become evident until several years later when the meniscus is progressively damaged.

Symptoms:

- The onset of symptoms is gradual.
- The person feels pain on the inner side of the knee joint during sports.
- The person feels pain when pressing on the joint line on the inner side of the knee.
- The joint may lock or click (caused by the torn portion of the meniscus catching on the end of the thighbone).
- A sports doctor trying to make the diagnosis of a meniscus injury will look for one or more of the signs listed below. If three or more of these signs are present, it is almost certain that the athlete has a meniscus tear:

    —Point tenderness when pressure is exerted on the joint line on the inner side of the knee

    —Pain in the joint line on the inner side of the knee when the knee is hyperflexed

    —Weakened or atrophied quadriceps muscle

    —Pain and a "clunk" sound when the foot and lower leg is turned and the bent knee is simultaneously straigthened. Known as the McMurray Test, pressure is applied to the knee and the leg is rotated internally and externally as illustrated in the following figure.

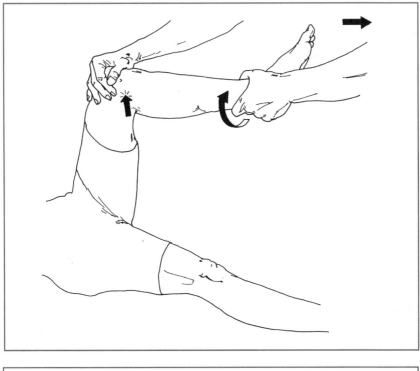

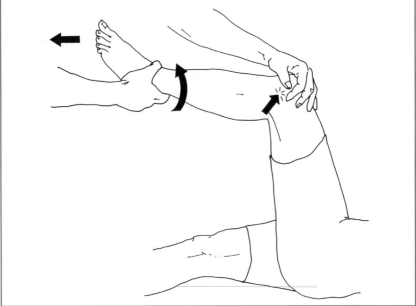

The McMurray Test

- Note: If the pain and symptoms described are felt on the outside of the knee, then there may be a lateral meniscus tear.

Concerns:

- Since blood supply to the meniscus is very poor, an injury to the meniscus will almost never heal itself. A runner with a damaged meniscus who wants to continue running will usually have to undergo surgery.
- Left untreated, a torn meniscus may worsen to the point where the entire meniscus has to be removed, instead of being repaired as described below.

Treatment:

What you can do

- Suspend running schedule, but do not completely discontinue exercise (see "Rehabilitation").
- Seek medical attention.
- If three or more of the symptoms are present (have a friend perform the test), begin a program of strengthening exercises to condition the quadriceps and hamstrings in anticipation of surgery and a subsequent layoff from running. Be sure the exercises do not worsen the damage— exercise within the pain threshold.
- For relief of minor to moderate pain, take acetaminophen or ibuprofen as label-directed, or for the relief of pain *and* inflammation, take aspirin if tolerated.

What the doctor can do

- The doctor will confirm the diagnosis through a physical examination and medical history (occasionally, the doctor may use an arthroscope to look inside the joint if he or she cannot make a definitive diagnosis).
- If the doctor cannot confirm the injury, he or she may order an MRI of the knee, which usually provides an excellent view of the meniscus.
- The doctor may recommend surgery and prescribe a preoperative conditioning program for the quadriceps.
- To repair a torn meniscus, the doctor usually performs a partial menisectomy. The doctor makes two small puncture holes in the

joint, places an arthroscope in one of the holes to look at the joint, and uses surgical instruments in the other hole to trim off the damaged portion of the meniscus. The wound requires only two or three stitches. The patient is released from the hospital the same day as the operation and is walking the next day with the use of crutches.
- Occasionally, if the tear is very small (within the four to five millimeter "red zone" around the edge of the meniscus), it can be repaired by microscopic stitching.
- Total surgical removal of the meniscus is no longer done, thanks to the emergence of arthroscopic technology.

Rehabilitation:

- Since surgery is almost always required to overcome this condition, the runner should immediately begin a strengthening program for the muscles in front and in back of the thigh (quadriceps and hamstrings) to ensure optimal quicker postoperative recovery.
- After arthroscopic surgery to repair a meniscus, begin rehabilitation exercises to strengthen the quadriceps and hamstrings within one to two days under the supervision of a physical therapist. After one week, the patient will be able to begin doing more vigorous rehabilitation exercises, accompanied by gentle stationary biking.

Recovery time:

After arthroscopic surgery to repair a torn meniscus, the athlete can usually expect to return to activities that put rotational stress on the knee joint within four to eight weeks.

The runner should continue to do strengthening exercises for the muscles of the thigh after returning to running.

OSGOOD-SCHLATTER SYNDROME

(Inflammation at the point where the kneecap tendon attaches to the top of the larger shinbone.)

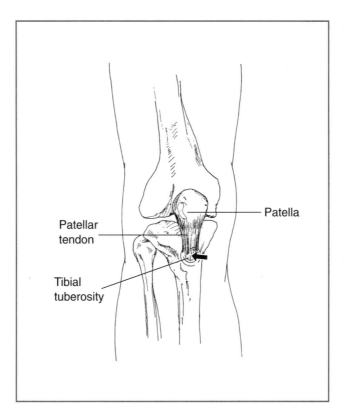

A child who has pain directly over the point where his or her kneecap tendon attaches to the shinbone may have Osgood-Schlatter syndrome, sometimes called Osgood-Schlatter disease.

This condition occurs for two reasons. First, the ends of children's bones are still growing and have not yet fully hardened. The softness at the ends of the growing bones predisposes them to damage from the tissues that attach to these areas, which tug at this vulnerable growing bone. Second, during growth spurts, children's bones grow faster than the muscle-tendons do, which makes the muscle-tendons tighter and more likely to pull on the point where they attach to bone.

Intensive sports activity involving running usually causes this condition, though it is more likely to occur in children between the ages of 9 and 14. It was previously thought that boys were more likely to develop Osgood-Schlatter syndrome, but with the emergence of girls in high school sports, it is now believed that this condition is not more common in one gender than the other.

Symptoms:

- The onset of symptoms is gradual and begins as a low-grade ache when the child gets out of bed in the morning, which worsens over the course of two weeks.
- Pain is felt directly over the point where the tendon attaches to the top of the front of the shin bone.
- The child will eventually be unable to run at full speed and may walk with a limp.
- The pain is especially acute when squatting, climbing stairs, or walking uphill.

Concerns:

- Ten percent of the athletes who sustain this condition develop a piece of bone in the tendon (ossicle) that can cause them pain throughout life.

Treatment:

What you can do

- Have the child administer ice massage, in conjunction with a "horseshoe pad" to relieve the pain.
- Take the child to a sports doctor.

What the doctor can do

- The doctor should refer the child to a physical therapist for a comprehensive strength and flexibility program that should correct this condition.
- The doctor should recommend that the child abstain from strenuous running activities during growth spurts.
- If X rays reveal that a free piece of bone has developed within the tendon, it may have to be removed through surgery if pain continues.

Rehabilitation:

When the initial symptoms abate, the child should participate in a conditioning program that stresses stretching the muscles in front and in back of the thigh (quadriceps and hamstrings). The child should do these stretching exercises with the kneecap taped or braced to reduce its movement and possible aggravation of the condition.

Recovery time:

This condition may take between two to four weeks and three years to resolve.

OSTEOCHONDRITIS DISSECANS OF THE KNEE

Knee

(A small divot in the surface of the knee joint that may eventually break off and fall into the joint)

If you have vague but acute pain when you run that feels as if it is *inside* the knee joint, and your knee sometimes locks, you may have osteochondritis dissecans.

In a manner similar to that found in the ankle, the grinding together of the ends of the bones that meet to form the knee joint causes this condition. Such friction can create a small crater with pieces of loose bone and cartilage around it, like a divot in the ground caused by a missed golf stroke. If the stress continues, chips of bone and cartilage may break off and fall into the joint.

In adults, bumping together of the ends of the bones may cause divots, though it is rare that pieces of bone and cartilage dislodge and fall into the joint. But in children, whose joint surfaces are much softer because they are made up of not-yet-hardened growing bone, there is a much greater chance that a portion of bone and cartilage can dislodge and fall into the joint. Children between the ages of 12 and 16 are especially at risk.

Symptoms:

Onset of symptoms is gradual. Loosening of the bone causes pain, and it is especially acute when the knee is used dynamically. The pain is nonspecific, though athletes occasionally describe it as being inside the joint. Pain abates after sports activity.

If a piece of bone and cartilage has dislodged and falls into the joint, the joint may occasionally lock. The athlete will be unable to fully straighten the injured knee.

Concerns:

If ignored, an osteochondritis dissecans without bone and cartilage dislodgment that could heal with rest will usually deteriorate to where a piece of this hard tissue dislodges and falls into the joint, which will inevitably require surgery.

Treatment:

What you can do

- A person with the symptoms described above should consult a sports doctor.
- Suspend running schedule, but do not completely discontinue exercise (see "Rehabilitation").
- For relief of minor to moderate pain, take acetaminophen or ibuprofen as label-directed, or for the relief of pain *and* inflammation, take aspirin if tolerated.

What the doctor can do

- The medical history will usually reveal if there is a loose or detached piece of joint cartilage.
- If the condition is severe and a piece of joint cartilage has broken off, the patient will complain of locking in the knee three or four times a day, and it will be difficult to fully straighten the leg. Just touching the joint will cause pain.
- To confirm the diagnosis of osteochondritis dissecans in the knee, as well as assess its severity, the doctor may order X rays of *both* knee joints. The view inside the uninjured knee provides a comparison to determine the bone cartilage displacement on the injured side. What is normally seen is either a piece of bone cartilage about to dislodge with further activity, or pieces that have already broken off.
- Because X rays do not allow doctors to see the actual joint surface, which is made of cartilage, sometimes they use an MRI or arthrogram to get a better look at the damage. These diagnostic tools allow doctors to examine the actual joint surface and, if the piece of joint cartilage has not yet detached, see the outline of the loose piece lying in its crater.

- Adults who have osteochondritis dissecans usually require surgery to repair the damaged joint. (In children, immobilization and rest usually allow the body's healing process to help the loose chip fully rejoin the joint. Three months of limited activity is usually necessary.)
- The surgical options are as follows:

  —The surgeon will make two puncture holes in the skin over the knee, and, using an arthroscope, will enter the joint and remove the loose piece of joint cartilage from the crater. The surgeon will make several tiny holes in the crater with a bone drill. The blood supply created by these drilled holes creates hard scar tissue.
  —Occasionally, the surgeon may pin the loose piece of bone back in place. If the initial diagnosis reveals that the injury has already deteriorated to where a bone chip has come loose, the piece of bone may be pinned back in place or, more commonly, removed arthroscopically. If the chip has lodged in a portion of the joint where an arthroscope cannot reach, the surgeon will make an incision over the knee and remove the chip.

- Treatment for osteochondritis dissecans depends on whether the piece of bone and cartilage has detached. If it has not, three to six months of relative rest may enable the divot to heal.

Rehabilitation:

- If relative rest is used to treat this condition, engage in cardiovascular exercise while waiting for it to heal. Do exercise that does not aggravate the condition, such as swimming, and, making allowances for the injured area, continue as usual with strength and flexibility conditioning.
- If the piece of bone and cartilage is simply removed and drilling is done, rehabilitation exercises can start within five days of surgery.
- If a fragment of bone is pinned back in place, the patient should keep weight off the knee for six weeks, though rehabilitation exercises can start in three weeks.

Recovery time:

- If nonoperative treatment is used, it may be three to six months before the patient can return to his or her full running schedule.
- When the fragment is removed and the crater is drilled, it will be 6 weeks before the patient can return to running.

- If the fragment has to be pinned in place, the runner can return to his or her schedule in 8 to 12 weeks.

Knee   PATELLOFEMORAL PAIN SYNDROME

(A variety of disorders centering on the kneecap.)

If you have pain in front of one or both kneecaps when you run, pain that abates after running but which worsens when you sit for extended periods or when walking up stairs, you may have patellofemoral pain syndrome.

Until recently, doctors usually diagnosed pain in the area of the knee-cap as chondromalacia patella. From the Greek *chondros* and *malakia*, this translates as "cartilage softness," in this case behind the kneecap. The term was coined at the turn of the century to describe actual damage to the back surface of the kneecap discovered during open surgery. Repetitive rubbing of the back surface of the kneecap on the thighbone usually caused the damage (disease or degeneration associated with aging may also cause this condition).

Unfortunately, subsequent generations of doctors began assuming that any athlete with these symptoms had chondromalacia patella. But we now know that athletes with these classic symptoms do not necessarily have damage to the back surface of the kneecap, and furthermore, that damage to the back surface of the kneecap does not necessarily mean a person will develop knee pain. Most significantly, we now know that treating chondromalacia patella surgically often does not clear up knee pain.

It is now clear that the diagnosis of chondromalacia patella was overused. Several conditions quite unrelated to damage to the back surface of the kneecap may cause kneecap pain. For this reason, athletes should beware the doctor who diagnoses their knee pain as chondromalacia patella unless he or she has detected damage to the back surface of the kneecap through an arthrotomy, arthroscopy, CAT scan, or MRI. Unless they have detected true chondromalacia, doctors now diagnose problems accompanied by the classic symptoms as patellofemoral pain syndrome.

An intensive running schedule usually precipitates patellofemoral pain syndrome, though it is more likely to occur if one or more of the following risk factors exist:

INTRINSIC   Anatomical abnormalities—Flat feet, thighs that turn inward from the hip, knock knees that create a Q angle greater than 15 or 20 degrees (see page 13), high-riding kneecaps (patella alta), a shallow thighbone groove in which the kneecap lies, looseness of the quadriceps tendon, or "miserable malalignment syndrome" (a combination of three of the above abnormalities—inward turning thighs, knock knees, and flat feet).

Poor conditioning or muscle imbalances—Hamstring muscles that are comparatively stronger and tighter than the quadriceps, or muscle on the outer side of the quadriceps (vastus lateralis) that is stronger than the one on the inside (vastus medialis).

EXTRINSIC   Training error—Excessively increasing the frequency, intensity, or duration of the running regimen.

Improper footwear—Worn-out shoes.

Symptoms:

- Onset of symptoms is gradual.
- Usually, the person feels pain in front of the kneecap and frequently in both kneecaps.
- The pain may be spread out, or localized along the inner or outer edge of the kneecap.
- The pain intensifies during sports activity and abates when the knee is not being used in sports.
- Typically, pain develops when the person with this condition sits for extended periods with the knee bent, as in a movie theater or during a long car ride, or when the person walks down stairs or downhill.
- Usually there is no swelling, although there may be occasional puffiness in the knee.
- There may be a crunching, crackling sensation in the knee that can actually be heard. This is known as crepitus.
- The athlete may complain of the knee giving way.
- The symptoms usually become progressively worse, or intensify and abate depending on sports activity levels.
- Instability of the kneecap would not indicate a pain syndrome, but an instability syndrome.

Concerns:

- Unless the athlete seeks competent sports medicine consultation to diagnose and treat this troublesome condition, it is unlikely to clear up.

Treatment:

What you can do

- Suspend running schedule, but do not completely discontinue exercise (see "Rehabilitation").
- For relief of minor to moderate pain, take acetaminophen or ibuprofen as label-directed, or for the relief of pain _and_ inflammation, take aspirin if tolerated.
- Seek the most expert form of sports medicine attention available.

What the doctor can do

- After ascertaining the exact cause of pain through physical examination in conjunction with diagnostic techniques such as X rays, arthrography, a CAT scan, an MRI, or a bone scan, the doctor may recommend or prescribe

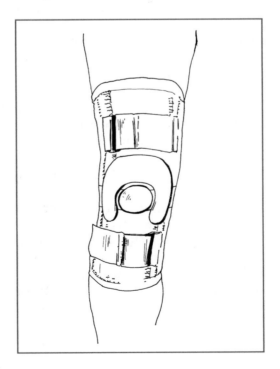

—anti-inflammatories to reduce pain and swelling,

—physical therapy (if the cause of the condition is imbalances in strength or flexibility),

—orthotics (if the cause is anatomical imbalances), or

—a knee brace (if the cause of the pain is erratic tracking of the kneecap).

- In about 10 to 20 percent of cases of patellofemoral pain syndrome, nonsurgical treatment fails and pain persists.
- Previously, it was thought that continuing pain was caused by damage to the back surface of the kneecap—true chondromalacia patella—and surgery was done to smooth the area. However, it has since been discovered that it is not chondromalacia patella that is primarily responsible for the pain, and surgery to repair the damage is not recommended.
- When surgery is done to correct pain in the kneecap, the major goal is not to repair damage to the back of the kneecap, but to relieve pressure that pulls the kneecap to the outside. In the procedure, known as a lateral retinacular release, the doctor cuts the connective tissues that are pulling the kneecap to the outside; sometimes, the doctor tightens up the muscles on the inside of the thigh that attach to the kneecap.

Rehabilitation:

- Engage in cardiovascular exercise that does not aggravate the condition, such as swimming, and, making allowances for the injured area, continue as usual with strength and flexibility conditioning.
- Engage in a flexibility program for the entire lower extremities. If pain persists for more than two weeks, consult a certified sports doctor (see pages 83-86). The doctor may prescribe an exercise program to alleviate muscle imbalances or strength and flexibility deficits that may be the underlying causes of the condition. The rehabilitation exercises may be supervised by a physical therapist or done independently. Particular attention should be paid to stretching the muscles in front, in back, and on the side of the thigh (quadriceps, hamstrings, and iliotibial band), and strengthening the muscles in front of the thigh (quadriceps) using straight leg raises (see pages 42-43).

Recovery time:

Whether treated with surgery or not, this condition takes between 6 and 12 weeks to resolve.

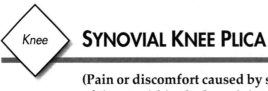

SYNOVIAL KNEE PLICA

(Pain or discomfort caused by snapping of specific bands of tissue within the knee joint, known as synovial plicae, between the edge of the thighbone and the kneecap.)

If you have a semilocking sensation in your knee, feel a snapping when you bend your knee past 15 or 20 degrees, and feel pain when sitting or squatting, you may have a synovial knee plica. This condition is very difficult to identify, however, because the symptoms mimic the symptoms of other knee disorders.

The cause of the symptoms is usually snapping of the plica over the end of the thighbone, which can cause roughening of the end of the thighbone and the underside of the kneecap.

Runners who train intensively may experience synovial knee plica conditions, although their cause is usually an excessively tight and unyielding plica.

Symptoms:

- This condition is difficult to identify, because the symptoms mimic the symptoms of other knee disorders.
- The athlete may experience a semilocking mechanism in the knee, and a snapping may be felt when the knee is bent past 15 or 20 degrees (these symptoms mimic those of a torn meniscus).
- There may be pain going up and down the stairs or when squatting.
- There is little or no swelling, and the joint is not loose.

Concerns:

- This condition is difficult to identify.

Treatment:

What you can do

- Suspend running schedule, but do not completely discontinue exercise (see "Rehabilitation").
- Use RICE, and consult a sports doctor.

What the doctor can do

- The doctor confirms the diagnosis through a process of elimination—by ruling out all other overuse knee conditions. Sometimes the plica can be felt on the inner edge of the kneecap.

- The doctor should attempt to treat the condition nonsurgically using rest and ice.
- If this does not work, and the condition recurs, it may be necessary to remove the plica surgically for the patient to resume problem-free running.

Rehabilitation:

- Engage in cardiovascular exercise that does not aggravate the condition, and, making allowances for the injured area, continue as usual with strength and flexibility conditioning.
- Engage in a flexibility program for the entire lower extremities. If pain persists for more than two weeks, consult a certified sports doctor (see pages 83-86). The doctor should prescribe an exercise program to alleviate muscle imbalances or strength and flexibility deficits that may be the underlying causes of the condition. The rehabilitation exercises may be supervised by a physical therapist or done independently. Particular attention should be paid to stretching the muscles on the outside of the thigh (iliotibial band) and strengthening the muscles in front of the thigh (quadriceps) using straight leg raises.
- When physical therapy is used to correct this condition, rehabilitation exercises should begin as soon as pain allows.

After surgery to remove the plica, rehabilitation exercises can begin within three to five days of the procedure.

Recovery time:

This condition may be resolved in four to six weeks, whether it is treated nonoperatively or surgically.

Hip, Pelvis, and Groin Injuries

Overuse injuries of the hip, pelvis, and groin area are caused by the repetitive contraction of the powerful muscle-tendon units in the area and the repetitive stress from the frequent pounding of the lower extremities on the running surface, which can carry up to the hip, pelvis, and groin area.

Overuse hip, pelvis, and groin injuries include bursitis and tendinitis conditions, stress fractures, and a unique inflammatory condition called osteitis pubis that affects the disk of cartilage between the right and left sides of the pubic bone.

In the pelvis and hip, the most commonly injured bursa sacs are the ischial, iliopectineal, and trochanteric bursae.

Irritation from repetitive muscle contractions usually causes these bursa conditions in runners. Fortunately, bursitis conditions in the hip and pelvis are rarely serious and seldom debilitating. They respond quite well to rest, anti-inflammatories, ice, and cortisone injections.

Inflammations of the muscle-tendon insertions into the bone are also seen in runners. Repetitive contractions of these muscle-tendon units cause the inflammations. Inflammations of the muscle-tendons—known as tendinitis—need to be differentiated from strains because they heal very differently. More severe cases may take an undetermined time to clear up and can be an extremely frustrating injury to resolve.

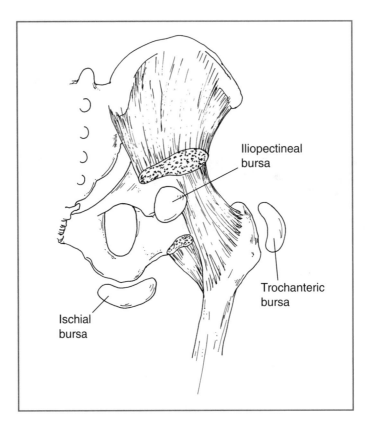

The most common tendinitis conditions in the hip, pelvis, and groin affect the adductor longus (the largest groin muscle), the iliopsoas (the largest hip flexor), and the rectus femoris (the main quadriceps muscle).

Stress fractures in the hip, pelvis, and groin area usually affect the pelvis or the femoral neck (the shaft of the thighbone just below the ball of the hip joint). Pelvic stress fractures are very rare, and are seen almost exclusively in elite distance runners. Even so, less than 2 percent of the stress fractures sustained by runners affect the pelvis.

More common are stress fractures of the femoral neck. Although this is technically an injury of the upper thigh, the runner usually experiences pain in the hip or groin as a nonspecific ache during and after activities using the hip.

A growing problem among distance runners is a condition known as osteitis pubis, an inflammation of the disk of cartilage where the right and left parts of the pubic bone meet. A runner with this condition experiences tenderness in the pubic bone that may radiate into the groin area.

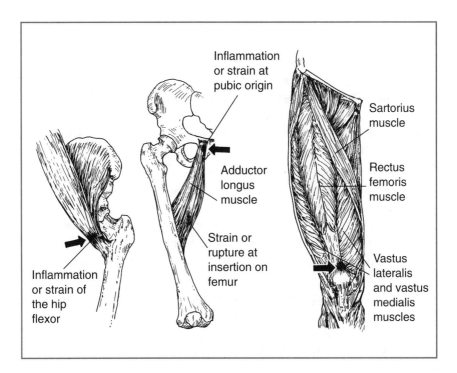

Inflammation or strain at pubic origin

Sartorius muscle

Adductor longus muscle

Rectus femoris muscle

Strain or rupture at insertion on femur

Inflammation or strain of the hip flexor

Vastus lateralis and vastus medialis muscles

Male Runners and Jock Itch

Jock itch, or tinea cruris, is a frequent complaint among male runners; it rarely affects their female counterparts. Characteristic symptoms include itchy, red, scaly patches on the groin, thighs, and buttocks. Pus-filled blisters may also develop.

Poor hygiene, inadequate ventilation of the groin area, and friction are the primary causes of jock itch. If left untreated, this condition can become chronic, spreading to the thighs and torso.

Prime candidates for jock itch are runners who wear an athletic supporter (jock strap), those who do not bathe soon after exercising, those who wear tight, constricting apparel or jockey shorts made of synthetic materials, those who are overweight, and those who have heavily muscled thighs that rub together during exercise.

(continued)

Proper hygiene, antifungal medication, and minimizing excessive warmth and moisture in the groin area are the fundamentals of treatment for this condition.

Gently wash the affected area with soap and water, making sure to rinse the soap completely to prevent irritation. Dry the area thoroughly. Twice daily apply a thin coating of over-the-counter clotrimazole (Lotrimin). Results should be seen in three to five days. Continue to use the medication for three to five days after the condition clears up. For several weeks, use a cornstarch-free powder (Zeasorb AF) after showering to keep the groin dry.

After running, do not linger in damp clothing. Wear loose fitting boxer shorts as underwear and change it daily. Always wear clean athletic clothing for exercise—especially shorts and undergarments. Overweight runners who sweat heavily and whose thighs rub together should lose weight. If these measures are unsuccessful, consult a dermatologist.

The doctor should use a scalpel to remove a tiny sample from the area. Examination under a microscope should reveal the exact cause of the condition.

To clear up the condition the doctor will usually recommend continuing the above regimen, and will usually prescribe oral antifungal medication, generally ketoconazole (Nizoral), or griseofulvin (Fulvicin-U/F, Gris-PEG, Grifulvin V) if the condition is a dermatophyte (such as ringworm or eczema). Almost always, such treatment will clear up the jock itch.

An intensive running schedule usually causes hip, pelvis, and groin overuse injuries, but intrinsic risk factors such as poor conditioning, muscle imbalances, or anatomical abnormalities may also cause injury.

Tightness in both the fascia lata, the wide portion at the top of the iliotibial band that crosses the outside of the hip, and the hamstrings, the group of muscles behind the thigh, is responsible for trochanteric bursitis, an inflammation of the bursa sac that lies over the hip joint. Anatomical imbalances such as flat feet, feet that turn inward (pronate) when the athlete runs, and unequal leg length may also precipitate trochanteric bursitis.

Another significant intrinsic risk factor for overuse injuries in the hip area is nutritional abuse. This risk factor is associated exclusively with the occurrence of stress fractures in women. Many women who train intensively and suffer from eating disorders may stop menstruating regularly. Irregular menstruation may cause these women's bones to lose density. When exposed to the repetitive demands of exercise, especially running, such bones are susceptible to stress fractures. The most frequent sites of these stress fractures are the bones of the foot and lower leg, although an increased incidence of stress fractures is being seen in the hip area, especially at the top of the thighbone just below the ball of the hip joint. For more information on the predisposition of some female runners to stress fractures, see chapter 10, "Special Concerns for Female Runners."

Extrinsic risk factors usually involved in hip, pelvis, and groin area injuries are training errors and inappropriate workout structure. (For a general discussion of intrinsic and extrinsic risk factors involved in overuse running injuries, see chapter 1; injury prevention guidelines can be found in chapter 2.)

OSTEITIS PUBIS

Hip,
Pelvis,
Groin

(Inflammation of the disk of cartilage [symphysis] that connects the right and left parts of the pubic bone.)

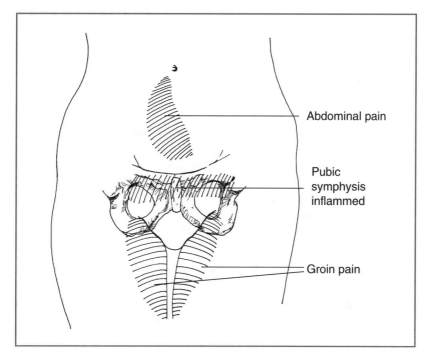

- Abdominal pain
- Pubic symphysis inflammed
- Groin pain

If you have pain in the front and center of your groin area radiating into the groin area, and this pain increases when you raise your leg outward or draw your leg inward against resistance, you may have osteitis pubis.

Though the exact cause of osteitis pubis is unknown, it usually occurs as a result of repetitive contraction of the muscles on the inner side of the thigh that attach to the pubic bone and the pubic symphysis. Osteitis pubis is more common in runners who have recently had prostate or bladder surgery.

Symptoms:

- Onset of symptoms is gradual.
- The runner feels pain and tenderness in the front and center of the pubic bone.
- Pain may radiate into the groin and into the inside of the thighs or the abdomen.
- Raising the leg outward and trying to draw it inward against resistance causes specific pain.
- As the condition worsens, pain increases, causing spasm in the abdominal muscles in the stomach and in the muscles on the inside of the thigh.

Concerns:

- If allowed to deteriorate, this condition will result in chronic pain in the groin.

Treatment:

What you can do

- Suspend running schedule, but do not completely discontinue exercise (see "Rehabilitation").
- For relief of minor to moderate pain, take acetaminophen or ibuprofen as label-directed, or for the relief of pain *and* inflammation, take aspirin if tolerated.
- Consult a sports doctor.

What the doctor can do

- The doctor may order X rays or bone scans to confirm the diagnosis.
- Nonsurgical treatment is usually used to correct this condition, and the doctor may prescribe rest and anti-inflammatories or a cortisone injection.

- If the condition has not been resolved after two to three months, surgery may be done to remove bone spurs on the symphysis.

Rehabilitation:

- Engage in nonweightbearing cardiovascular exercise that does not aggravate the condition, such as swimming and stationary biking, and, making allowances for the injured area, continue as usual with strength and flexibility conditioning.
- Engage in a flexibility program for the entire lower extremities. If pain persists for more than two weeks, consult a certified sports doctor (see pages 83-86). The doctor should prescribe an exercise program to alleviate muscle imbalances or strength and flexibility deficits that may be the underlying causes of the condition. The rehabilitation exercises may be supervised by a physical therapist or done independently. Particular attention should be paid to strengthening the stomach muscles that attach to the pelvis (abdominals), and stretching and strengthening the muscles in the groin area (adductor longus, adductor magnus, pectineus).

Recovery time:

- It may take between two and six months for this condition to be resolved.
- After surgery, the athlete can return to a strenuous running schedule within four to six weeks.

STRESS FRACTURES AT THE TOP OF THE THIGHBONE

(A series of tiny cracks in the thighbone just below the ball of the hip joint.)

If you have persistent pain in the groin and outside the thigh that sometimes extends down to the knee, limited hip motion, and pain when pushing on the hip bone, you may have a stress fracture at the very top of the thighbone.

Repetitive microtrauma in the lower extremities transmitted to the top of the thighbone causes this condition.

Stress fractures usually occur as a result of an intensive running schedule, though they are more likely to occur if one or more of the following risk factors exist:

INTRINSIC　Nutritional abuse - Women who menstruate irregularly because of poor diet and excessive exercise often develop bone thinning, and are therefore at increased risk of stress fractures.

EXTRINSIC　Training errors - Rapid increases in the frequency, intensity, and duration of the running regimen.

Symptoms:

- Onset of symptoms is gradual, but eventually, persistent pain is felt in the groin and the outside of the thigh, sometimes extending down to the knee.
- The runner may walk with a limp.
- There is limited hip motion, especially when turning the leg inward.
- There is minimal tenderness because of the depth of the overlying muscle. However, the runner may feel pain when pushing on the hip bone.

Concerns:

- In children, stress fractures at the top of the thighbone may interrupt blood supply to the ball of the hip joint, causing it to "die" (avascular necrosis).
- If allowed to worsen, a stress fracture can lead to a complete fracture.

Treatment:

What you can do

- Suspend running schedule, but do not discontinue exercise entirely.
- Use crutches if pain is severe.
- For relief of minor to moderate pain, take acetaminophen or ibuprofen as label-directed, or for the relief of pain *and* inflammation, take aspirin if tolerated.
- Consult a sports doctor.

What the doctor can do

- Because of the potential for severe disability if the bone becomes displaced, the doctor must be highly skeptical.

- The doctor should order X rays or a bone scan to try to confirm the diagnosis. Even if the stress fracture does not show up on X rays and symptoms persist (stress fractures often do not show until two or four weeks after initial symptoms are felt), the doctor should assume there is stress fracture.
- If the stress fracture cannot be seen on the initial X rays, the doctor will usually order another set of X rays or bone scans two to four weeks after the first X rays are taken.
- Initial care for this injury is relative rest. The athlete should use crutches for six or more weeks and begin strengthening exercises as soon as possible.
- X rays may be taken weekly to monitor the injury.

Rehabilitation:

- Engage in nonweightbearing cardiovascular exercise that does not aggravate the condition, such as swimming, and, making allowances for the injured area, continue as usual with strength and flexibility conditioning.
- After the fracture has healed and pain is gone, engage in a flexibility program for the entire lower extremities. Begin a prescribed exercise program to alleviate muscle imbalances or strength and flexibility deficits that may be the underlying causes of the condition. The rehabilitation exercises may be supervised by a physical therapist or done independently. Particular attention should be paid to general conditioning of the lower extremities while healing takes place. The focus should be on stretching the muscles in front of the hip (psoas), in back of the thigh (hamstrings), and the calf and heel cord area in back of the lower leg (gastro-soleus/Achilles tendon unit), because tightness in these areas may interfere with foot strike, therefore transmitting excessive stress to the thighbone.

Recovery time:

It may take two or more months to resolve this condition.

TROCHANTERIC BURSITIS

(An inflammation of the bursa sac that lies over the hip joint.)

If you have pain and a snapping sensation over the bony prominence on the outside of the hip, and the pain becomes especially acute when you move the leg of the affected side away from the body, you may have trochanteric bursitis.

This condition is caused by repetitive contraction of the muscle over the hip bone, which in some circumstances may irritate the bursa sac between the muscle and the hip joint.

Trochanteric bursitis is usually precipitated by an intensive running schedule, though it is more likely to occur if one or more of the following risk factors exist:

INTRINSIC   Anatomical abnormalities—Flat feet, differences in leg length, wide pelvis (this condition is seen more often in female runners).

Poor conditioning or muscle imbalances—Tightness in the muscles over the hip.

EXTRINSIC   Training errors—Excessively increasing the frequency, intensity, or duration of running schedule.

Symptoms:

- The onset of symptoms is gradual.
- The runner feels pain over the bony prominence on the outside of the hip (at the top of the outside of the thigh).
- The pain is especially acute when attempting hip abduction (moving the leg away from the body in a sideways direction).
- Sometimes snapping is felt over the joint.
- The athlete may walk with a limp.
- As the condition worsens, pain may begin to radiate down the thigh, especially when sleeping.
- In its most severe manifestation, adhesions that develop within the bursa may create a creaking sound (crepitus) when the hip is used. These adhesions may be felt as a series of tiny bumps between the skin and bone.

Concerns:

This condition rarely resolves itself, so it is extremely important to seek medical assistance.

Treatment:

What you can do

- Suspend running schedule, but do not completely discontinue exercise (see "Rehabilitation").
- Use ice to reduce inflammation (ice massage is especially effective).
- For relief of minor to moderate pain, take acetaminophen or ibuprofen as label-directed, or for the relief of pain *and* inflammation, take aspirin if tolerated.
- Consult a sports doctor.

What the doctor can do

- Usually, treatment for this condition is nonsurgical. The doctor may recommend or prescribe

    —anti-inflammatories to reduce pain and swelling,
    —draining the bursa with a syringe,
    —a cortisone injection,
    —orthotics (if the cause of the condition is flat feet, feet that excessively pronate when running, or unequal leg length), or
    —physical therapy (if the cause of the condition is tightness in the muscles over the hip).

- If the condition has been allowed to become severe, surgical intervention may be necessary. In this procedure, the doctor will enter the joint and remove the adhesions that have developed in the bursa sac and will usually remove the bursa sac at the same time. Often, the doctor performs a release of the iliotibial band by cutting open the tissue so it does not rub the bursa.

Rehabilitation:

- Engage in cardiovascular exercise that does not aggravate the condition, such as swimming, and, making allowances for the injured area, continue as usual with strength and flexibility conditioning.
- Engage in a flexibility program for the entire lower extremities. If pain persists for more than two weeks, consult a certified sports doctor (see pages 83-86). The doctor should prescribe an exercise program to alleviate muscle imbalances or strength and flexibility deficits that may be the underlying causes of the condition. The rehabilitation exercises may be supervised by a physical therapist or done independently. Particular attention should be paid to stretching the iliotibial band that runs down the side of the thigh, the muscles on the outside of the hip (tensor fascia latae, gluteus

minimus, gluteus maximus), and the muscles that attach to the pelvis, especially those that rotate the hip outward. The runner should both stretch and strengthen the muscles on the outside of the hip.

Recovery time:

- When treated without surgery, this condition may be resolved in four to six weeks.
- Following surgery, it may take six or more weeks for this condition to be resolved.

Back Injuries

Chronic back pain is extremely common in Americans. Approximately 60 to 80 percent of all Americans develop low back pain at some point in their lives.

Runners are even more likely than sedentary people to develop lower back pain, especially those runners 30 and older. Running subjects the spine to continuous low-intensity stress—the back is flat when the foot strikes the ground, but bends slightly backward when the back foot leaves the ground. This repetitive stress is substantial. The faster a person runs, the more pronounced the bending and straightening motion becomes, and the more severe the stress.

Furthermore, running can cause muscle imbalances that predispose the runner to pain in the lower back. When done exclusively, running tends to strengthen and tighten the muscles in the lower back, the front of the hip, and behind the thigh, making them relatively stronger than their opposing muscles—the stomach, behind the hip, and the quadriceps. These imbalances can cause a postural malalignment in the back called swayback, in which there is an excessive front-to-back curve in the lower back. Some people are naturally swaybacked.

Runners with swayback are at increased risk of developing lower back pain. This postural abnormality puts the tissues in the lower back in a continuous position of overstretching, which may be exacerbated when the person runs. Back pain experienced by runners may also have a more serious origin: swayback may cause serious overuse conditions of the spinal structure such as a herniated disk or spondylolysis.

Overuse back injuries include conditions caused by repetitive low-intensity stress (especially excessive forward and backward bending), poor conditioning or muscle imbalances, anatomical abnormalities, bad posture, and degenerative conditions associated with aging.

Tightness and weakness in certain muscle groups can cause back problems. Besides swayback, anatomical abnormalities such as leg length differences or an uneven pelvis may also lead to back problems. A person with one leg longer than the other tends to run with the spine in a slight sideways curve. As a result, wear and tear may take place on the concave side of the spine if the person subjects the back to the stresses of running.

Sometimes a person is misdiagnosed as having one leg longer than the other when the person's pelvis is uneven. Having an uneven pelvis causes the same problems in running that a leg length discrepancy does—a slight sideways curve in the spine that causes wear and tear in the concave side when the person runs. Determining whether a person has an uneven pelvis requires that they undergo X rays.

Age is a risk factor that profoundly influences running injuries of the back, particularly problems affecting the disks. As a person gets older his or her disks degenerate, losing their resilience to the stress caused by running. For that reason, back problems associated with the disks, known colloquially as slipped disks, generally affect runners over 30 years old.

Extrinsic risk factors usually involved in overuse back injuries are training errors and an inappropriate workout structure. (For a general discussion of intrinsic and extrinsic risk factors involved in overuse running injuries, see chapter 1; injury prevention guidelines, as well as a program for conditioning the back, can be found in chapter 2.)

SLIPPED DISK/HERNIATED DISK/ RUPTURED DISK

Back

(Degeneration in the lower back disks that causes pressure on the nerves.)

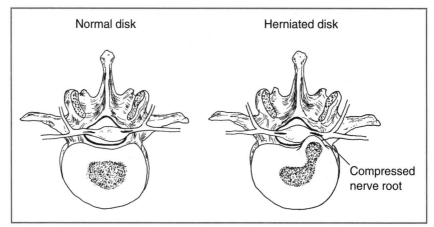

Normal disk   Herniated disk

Compressed nerve root

If you have pain, tingling, and numbness that radiate from your buttocks down one leg, you may have intervertebral disk disease, more commonly known as a slipped, herniated, or ruptured disk.

The natural degeneration of the disks that takes place in daily life and sports causes this condition. The cracks in the shell of the disk allows the pulp in the center of the disk to leak out and exert pressure on the large nerves in the area.

Intervertebral disk disease usually affects people over 20 years old, though it is more likely to occur if the following risk factors exist.

INTRINSIC Imbalances in muscle strength or flexibility—Running causes the lower back and hip flexor muscles to become stronger than their opposing muscles, the abdominal and hip extensor muscles; this in turn leads to a postural abnormality called swayback, which puts excessive stress on the lower back, including the disks.

Anatomical abnormalities—Swayback, a postural abnormality; uneven leg length; uneven pelvis.

EXTRINSIC Training error—Excessively increasing the intensity, frequency, or duration of training.

Symptoms:

- Pain, tingling, and numbness radiate from the buttocks down the leg, and in severe cases, all the way to the little toe. This is known as sciatica.
- There is muscle weakness in the affected limb, and the leg may give way.
- The pain worsens with coughing and straining.

Treatment:

What you can do

- Suspend running schedule, but do not completely discontinue exercise (see "Rehabilitation").
- Ice the back for the first 48 to 72 hours.
- Rest in bed in the *psoas* position (with the knees bent) until the pain dissipates.
- Use a moist heating pad to control muscle spasm.

- For relief of minor to moderate pain, take acetaminophen or ibuprofen as label-directed, or for the relief of pain *and* inflammation, take aspirin if tolerated.
- Begin an exercise program as soon as possible to strengthen the abdominal and lower back muscles.
- See a doctor if you have excruciating pain or sciatica (pain, tingling, and numbness radiating from the buttocks down the leg, and in severe cases, all the way to the little toe).
- Seek emergency medical attention if there is any change in bladder or bowel function.

What the doctor can do

- Nonsurgical treatment is most often used to manage this condition. The doctor may recommend or prescribe

  —continued abstention from running for 8 to 12 weeks, or until symptoms completely resolve, or
  —anti-inflammatories, traction, or cortisone injection.

- If the condition does not resolve itself after nonsurgical treatment and a wait-and-see period of three to six months, surgery may be considered.
- In the procedure, known as a diskectomy, the doctor makes an incision and removes the piece of disk that is compressing the nerve. No bracing is necessary after such surgery. The athlete should begin walking as soon as possible. When necessary, a diskectomy is a safe and successful method of correcting this troublesome problem.

Rehabilitation:

- When initial pain dissipates, begin an overall program to condition the back and other important structures. The focus should be on restoring flexibility in the lower back itself (lumbodorsal fascia), as well as in the muscles in front of the hip (psoas) and in back of the thigh (hamstrings). Strengthening of the stomach muscles (abdominals) should also be done.
- After surgery, begin rehabilitation exercises as soon as pain allows, preferably within three to five days.

Recovery time:

- Complete recovery is possible, but the runner may be subject to episodic pain, usually related to his or her activity level.

- Unless surgery is done to alleviate this problem, the condition is usually recurrent. Episodes may last anywhere between a day or so to several months.
- After surgery, the athlete should wait six to eight weeks before returning to full activity.

SPONDYLOLYSIS AND SPONDYLOLYSTHESIS 〈 *Back* 〉

(Spondylolysis is a stress fracture of the vertebra; spondylolysthesis is a stress fracture of the vertebra that also involves slippage of a portion of the vertebra.)

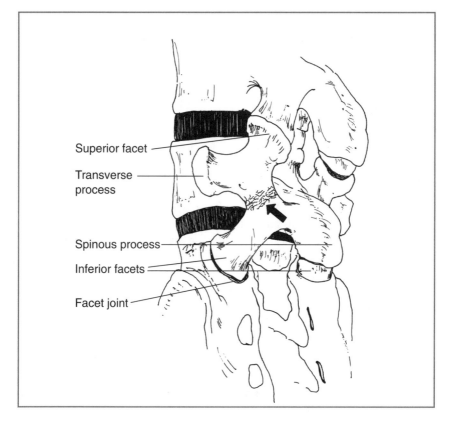

Superior facet

Transverse process

Spinous process

Inferior facets

Facet joint

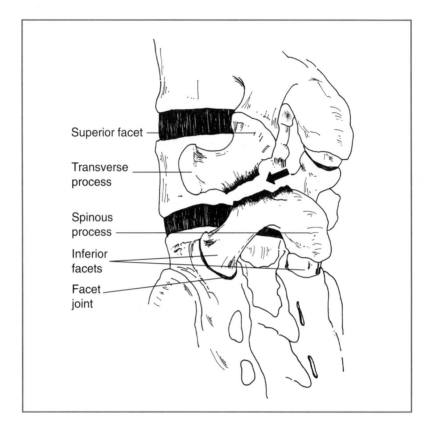

Superior facet

Transverse
process

Spinous
process

Inferior
facets

Facet
joint

If you have general lower back pain and stiffness in one or both sides, and have difficulty bending backward, you may have either spondylolysis or spondylolysthesis.

The repetitive low-intensity, forward- and backward-bending motion that may occur during running stresses a particular area in the lower back and causes these conditions.

An intensive running schedule may precipitate this condition, though it is more likely to occur if one or more of the following risk factors exist.

INTRINSIC   Anatomical abnormalities—Swayback (abnormally large front-to-back curvature in the lower spine), thinness of the vertebrae.

Poor conditioning or muscle imbalances—Running develops the muscles of the lower back, front of the hip, and back of the thigh, causing them to become stronger and tighter than their opposing muscles, those in the stomach, back of the hip, and front of the thigh; this in turn may lead to swayback.

EXTRINSIC   Training errors—Excessively increasing the frequency, duration, or intensity of training.

Symptoms:

- Onset of symptoms is gradual.
- The runner feels general lower back pain and stiffness on one or both sides.
- Bending forward or backward is difficult and painful.
- Pain, tingling, and numbness radiate from the buttocks down the leg, and in severe cases, all the way to the little toe. This condition, known as sciatica, may involve muscle weakness in the affected limb that may cause the leg to give way.

Concerns:

- Unless spondylolysis is caught in its early stages and treated properly, it is likely to cause episodic back pain.

Treatment:

What you can do

- Suspend running schedule, as well as any other activities that involve bending backward (avoid sit-ups, weightlifting, etc.). However, do not completely discontinue exercise (see "Rehabilitation").
- Wear an elastic back brace (available at most drugstores).
- For relief of minor to moderate pain, take acetaminophen or ibuprofen as label-directed, or for the relief of pain *and* inflammation, take aspirin if tolerated.
- Consult a sports doctor.

What the doctor can do

- Usually, treatment for this condition is nonsurgical. The doctor may recommend or prescribe

  —anti-inflammatories to reduce pain and inflammation,
  —heat treatments,
  —a back brace to prevent bending that will aggravate the condition, or
  —physical therapy.

- In rare cases, when a vertebra has slipped more than 50 percent of the width of the vertebrae above and below it, or there is severe pain, surgery may be necessary. In this procedure, called a spinal fusion, a bony bridge is created between the solid sacrum at the bottom of the spine and the area of slippage. This fusion effectively prevents further slippage. Spinal fusion is an extremely safe and successful way to correct this condition.

Rehabilitation:

- The focus on rehabilitation for this condition is exercise to correct lordosis, or curvature of the spine. This is done by strengthening the stomach muscles (abdominals) and stretching the muscles in the front of the hip and in back of the thigh (hamstrings), as well as improving the overall flexibility of the spine.

- Begin rehabilitation exercises when pain allows.

Recovery time:

- Spondylolysis (stress fracture of the vertebra without slipping) is resolved after one week of rest.
- Mild to moderate spondylolysthesis (25 to 50 percent slippage of the vertebra) requires one to three months to resolve.
- After a surgical spinal fusion to correct severe spondylolysthesis, it will be six months before the athlete can return to full activity. At this time, however, the back is stronger than before.
- Without surgical treatment, the symptoms will probably recur.

Back ◇ **MECHANICAL LOWER BACK PAIN**

(If you have vague pain and stiffness in your lower back, sometimes accompanied by muscle spasm, you may have a chronic back condition known as mechanical lower back pain)

The precise cause of lower back pain is unknown, but it is a frequent condition in runners as well as in the general population. It is thought to be brought on by a combination of factors, including muscle strains, anatomical abnormalities, faulty posture, and poor physical conditioning.

An intensive running schedule may precipitate mechanical lower back pain, but it is more likely to occur if one or more of the following risk factors exist:

INTRINSIC   Previous injury—Because pain in the lower back often causes a person, consciously or unconsciously, to avoid using his or her back, the muscles important to maintaining lower back health weaken and tighten.

Anatomical abnormalities—Swayback.

Poor conditioning or muscle imbalances—Excessive strength and tightness in certain muscle groups, especially the lower back, the front of the hip, and the back of the thigh.

EXTRINSIC   Training error—Excessively hard running surface.

Symptoms:

- There is general pain and stiffness in the lower back, sometimes accompanied by muscle spasm.
- Motion is restricted.
- The pain does not radiate into the buttocks or legs (this is a sign of intervertebral disk disease, covered on pages 180-183).

Treatment:

What you can do

- Rest and ice the back in the initial stages of pain.
- Suspend running schedule, but do not completely discontinue exercise (see "Rehabilitation").
- For relief of minor to moderate pain, take acetaminophen or ibuprofen as label-directed, or for the relief of pain *and* inflammation, take aspirin if tolerated.
- Participate in a conditioning program to develop strength and flexibility in the tissues necessary for preventing lower back pain (see pages 45-50).

What the doctor can do

- The doctor should determine the exact cause of the lower back pain.
- The doctor can recommend a physical therapist who specializes in rehabilitating the condition.

Rehabilitation:

- Engage in cardiovascular exercise that does not aggravate the condition, such as swimming, stationary biking (in an upright posture), or using stairclimbing machines (use small steps on such machines), and, making allowances for the injured area, continue as usual with strength and flexibility conditioning.
- As soon as possible, begin an overall program to condition the back and other important structures. The focus should be on restoring flexibility in the lower back itself (lumbodorsal fascia), as well as in the muscles in front of the hip (psoas) and in back of the thigh (hamstrings). The stomach muscles (abdominals) should also be strengthened.
- After pain dissipates, begin the strength and flexibility program described in chapter 2.

Recovery time:

Although episodes of pain may recur, the initial symptoms usually dissipate after several days.

Special Concerns for Female Runners

Women in increasing numbers are participating and excelling in running. The road was paved for the emergence of top runners and recreational runners alike by the enormous increase in the participation of women in sports and fitness activities. Until quite recently, women were excluded from the sports milieu in the belief that they were not physically or emotionally equipped for its rigors. Women have traditionally been regarded as psychologically capricious, weaker than men, and more likely to become injured. In ancient Greece, women were not only prohibited from participating in the Olympic Games, they were not allowed to watch.

Attitudes began to change around the turn of the twentieth century, when women began taking up activities such as tennis, mountaineering, and skiing. Still, sports that involved strenuous exertion, physical contact, or intense competition—running included—remained out of bounds, because these activities were considered unladylike and dangerous for women.

An example of the traditional attitude toward women runners was the absence, until recently, of distance running events for women. In the 1928 Olympics, an 800-meter competition was added with only three weeks notice. The previous maximum distance for women was 300 meters! A number of the competitors were inadequately prepared and collapsed without finishing the race. The ensuing controversy set back women's distance running competition several decades.

Federal and state equal rights laws have sparked an explosion in sports participation among girls. Our schools are now required to provide equal access to sports facilities. The results have been dramatic. Not only are more girls taking part in traditional women's sports such as field hockey, basketball, gymnastics, tennis, and softball, but they are also making inroads into male sports bastions such as running. Legions

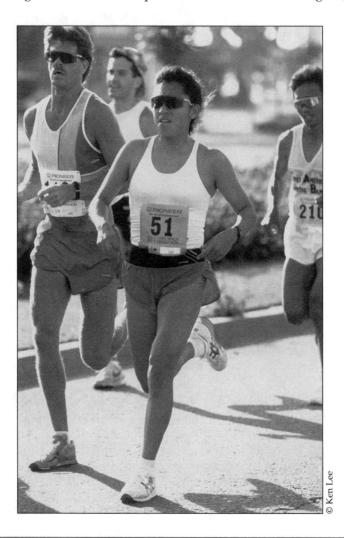

As more women have joined the competitive running ranks, negative myths surrounding their hardiness have disappeared.

of young women have been participating in running at the high school and college levels, and many of them continue running after their competitive days are over.

The fitness boom of the last decade has inspired women who had never participated in organized running to take to the streets in jogging suits and sneakers.

As increasing numbers of women began to participate in recreational and competitive sports, as well as in the Olympic games, negative myths and concerns about the hardiness of women dissolved. Following that trend came research into gender-specific elements of their participation. It quickly became clear that what was understood about men's sports performance could not simply be extrapolated to women. The following sections address special concerns of women runners.

The Female Athlete Triad: Eating Disorders, Menstrual Irregularities, and Stress Fractures

The relationship among three distinct but interrelated conditions—eating disorders, menstrual irregularities, and stress fractures—has puzzled sports professionals as long as women have participated in vigorous exercise. The sports medicine profession has only recently come to understand how these phenomena are interrelated. In 1993, an American College of Sports Medicine task force on the special problems of female athletes coined a term to describe the relationship: the female athlete triad.

Female athletes, especially runners, have more eating disorders than their sedentary counterparts. Poor eating habits combined with a high level of activity can cause a woman's body fat level to drop below the level necessary for normal menstrual function. The result is that women stop having their periods (amenorrhea), or have periods irregularly (oligomenorrhea), and in turn lose much of the estrogen necessary for bone-rebuilding that normal bodies perform on a continuous basis. This can cause premature osteoporosis and predispose an athlete to stress fractures.

Female runners and their family, friends, colleagues, and exercise partners should know of the potential serious consequences of this phenomenon, which may include death. The key to treating the female athlete triad is prevention and early intervention, made possible by education.

Eating Disorders Among Female Athletes

Disordered eating is a significant problem among female runners. Studies show that from 15 to 62 percent of female athletes have eating disorders severe enough to meet the criteria for anorexia nervosa and bulimia nervosa. By comparison, only 1 percent of the general female population meet these criteria. Moreover, the current research may underrepresent the problem. Although their behaviors may not fit the criteria for anorexia or bulimia, many female runners exhibit eating habits and nutritional status that put them at risk for developing serious psychiatric, endocrine, and skeletal problems.

Eating disorders are common among recreational athletes who engage in sports and exercise primarily for weight control, particularly runners and aerobic dancers. The female runner's focus on exercise, diet, and body composition may become an obsession when thinness

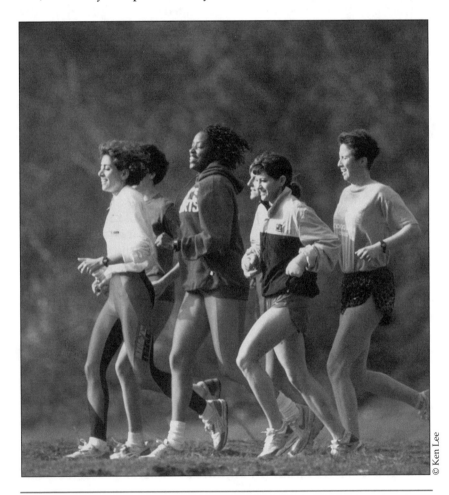

© Ken Lee

Female athletes exhibit a higher percentage of eating disorders than the general female population.

rather than health and fitness becomes the overriding objective. Many reach the point where no amount of running is enough, and no weight loss is too much.

The dangers of anorexia nervosa and bulimia nervosa in the general population are well known. These two eating disorders can lead to many psychiatric, endocrine, and orthopedic problems, that may, in their most extreme cases, cause death. Among anorexic nonathletes who do receive treatment, there is a mortality rate of between 10 and 18 percent. The sooner intervention starts, the better the chance for recovery.

Effects of Eating Disorders and Vigorous Exercise on Menstrual Regularity

Among the possible consequences of vigorous exercise and low body weight on menstruation are delay of menarche (when females begin having their periods), amenorrhea (when periods cease), and oligomenorrhea (when periods occur infrequently [fewer than six per year]).

Evidence suggests that one of the principal reasons women stop having their periods is that their body fat levels drop below a certain percentage of body mass (estimated at 17 percent). When body fat decreases, estrogens also decrease and androgens increase, which may result in menstrual irregularity.

Reflecting the relationship between menstrual irregularities and nutritional issues (of which eating disorders are a part), amenorrhea and oligomenorrhea are particularly prevalent among runners. (These conditions are also frequently seen in sports in which a lean physique and low body fat are considered to be advantageous, such as gymnastics, ballet dancing, and figure skating). Depending on which study is used, the reported incidence of amenorrhea in young female athletes ranges from 3.4 percent all the way up to 66 percent. In contrast, the reported prevalence of amenorrhea in the nonathletic female population is 2 percent to 5 percent.

There are factors other than low body fat levels, however, that may cause amenorrhea or oligomenorrhea. This explains why female athletes with normal body fat levels suffer menstrual irregularities more than the general population and why many female athletes with low body fat levels menstruate regularly.

Psychological stress is one such factor. Running for fun can lower stress, but at a competitive level running can be a source of heightened stress. Stress can cause a woman to stop menstruating. Other reasons may include pregnancy, hypothyroidism, pituitary adenoma, polycystic ovarian disease, and androgen excess syndromes.

Menarche refers to the time in her life when a female first starts having her periods. In the United States, the average age of menarche is between 12 and 13 years. Yet girls participating in sports such as running, gymnastics, ballet dancing, and figure skating may not start their periods until they are closer to 16 years of age. Again, the percentage of body weight as fat seems to be a key factor in determining the onset of menarche, as well as the psychological stress experienced by elite female athletes. The typical athlete who experiences delay in menarche is a young athlete who is driven to excel in her sport and who is obsessed with her appearance because she believes or has been told that performance is linked to thinness.

While it is understood that many female runners may suffer from amenorrhea or oligomenorrhea, what is not as well understood is whether there are dangers (besides skeletal injury risk) associated with menstrual irregularities. Until recently, when stress fracture concerns surfaced, it was thought that the dangers were minimal. In fact, many committed female runners found it desirable not to have the inconvenience of menstruating because it interfered with their running schedule. More significant, studies showed that athletes with menstrual irregularities had not experienced any long-term impairment of gynecological and reproductive function. A survey of 107 of the women champions in the 1952 Olympic Games found that none suffered permanent impairment. A 1972 study of former elite international female athletes revealed that these women had fewer complications during pregnancy and easier deliveries than either a group of normally active women or a less physically active group.

Usually periods resume after vigorous exercise is discontinued, and at that stage many women report favorable changes: lighter flow, less cramping and discomfort, and shorter duration of flow.

Menstrual Irregularity and Skeletal Injury Risk

Regular exercise is known to combat the effects of osteoporosis. In certain circumstances, however, exercise has been shown to hasten the onset of osteoporosis and increase the likelihood of conditions such as stress fractures.

Osteoporosis is a bone disease that causes bones to thin and weaken. Though osteoporosis can affect men, it is much more likely to affect women, especially after menopause. With osteoporosis, bone minerals—mainly calcium—are lost, and bones become so brittle that a minor injury can break a wrist, hip, or spine.

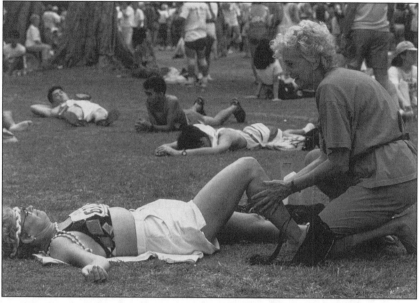

Diet and exercise play a role in the onset of premature osteoporosis and stress fractures in women.

Osteoporosis can occur in young women, too. Decreased estrogen levels associated with delayed menarche, oligomenorrhea, or amenorrhea can cause premature osteoporosis. Premature osteoporosis is often seen in very athletic young women who exercise or diet so strenuously their periods do not start, or, once started, become irregular, or cease altogether. Untreated, these young women may lose up to 20 percent of their skeletal mass, and may end up in their twenties with the bone density of a 50-year-old woman. Current research shows that bone loss is irreversible. Not only do these women lose bone mineral density and become osteoporotic, but they may never regain their previous bone densities.

Unlike older women with osteoporosis who are susceptible to complete fractures, younger women with menstrual irregularities are more likely to sustain stress fractures. Among young female athletes with amenorrhea, there is an almost tripled incidence of stress fractures. A study of female college athletes showed only 9 percent of those who regularly menstruated experienced stress fractures, as compared to 24 percent of athletes with irregular or no periods. The most common sites of stress fractures in female athletes are the back, hip, pelvis, lower leg, and foot.

Warning Signs of the Female Triad

Female athletes who exercise primarily for weight control must be wary of their susceptibility to disordered eating habits. Family members, friends, and colleagues should be vigilant. The typical athlete with an eating disorder is somewhat obsessive, introverted, reserved, self-denying, overcompliant, and rigid in her views.

If a woman answers "yes" to any of the following questions, she should seek medical counsel:

- Do you use or have you ever used laxatives? Diuretics? Diet pills?
- Have you ever made yourself vomit to lose weight or to get rid of a big meal?
- Do you skip meals or avoid certain foods?

In addition to direct questions about disordered eating such as the ones above, the medical professional may ask these questions:

- Have you lost weight recently? What weight-loss technique do you use?
- What is the most and the least you have weighed in the last year?
- What is your ideal weight?

The examining physician should be aware of the significance of the woman's menstrual status in foreshadowing potential problems. In taking a menstrual history, the doctor might ask these questions:

- When did you start having your period?
- How regular has it been?
- Have you ever missed any periods? How many months in a row? How many cycles per year?

Athletes with irregular periods require further assessment, including detailed questioning about nutrition, disordered eating habits, training intensity, and daily stress. Additional questions include the following:

(continued)

- How many hours per day and per week do you exercise?
- Do you take calcium supplements? How much dietary calcium do you take?
- Have you ever used birth control pills?
- Have you ever had a stress fracture or other fracture?

Though many female athletes do not show outward signs of the female triad, physicians should look for physical clues during the physical examination.

Women who restrict food intake may be quite thin, but those who binge and purge are often of normal weight or even slightly overweight.

Although athletes have a slower pulse rate than inactive people, a decreased pulse rate is one of the body's responses to disordered eating. A pulse rate of 40 to 50 beats per minute should raise the physician's index of suspicion.

Hypotension can also be a sign of an eating disorder. Patients may get light-headed from dehydration and electrolyte imbalances caused by their eating disorders. Hypothermia may also indicate disordered eating behavior and thermoregulatory abnormalities.

Other physical exam signs will indicate to the examining physician that the patient is hiding a more extreme disorder.

Facial hair, one of the body's responses to starvation, may indicate severe anorexia. Patients who have bulimia often have parotic gland swelling, or so-called chipmunk cheeks. It is important for doctors to examine the patient's mouth and teeth. Self-induced vomiting often causes erosion of tooth enamel. Patients who have bulimia have often had dental work, including root canals.

Stress fractures may be the ultimate tip-off of the female triad, especially when the female athlete sustains several stress fractures in a period of a year or two. Often, these athletes are amenorrheic and have eating disorders.

Treating the Female Triad

Treating the female triad is primarily a question of education and early intervention. Once the physician diagnoses the triad, he or she should enlist the services of a psychologist and nutritionist to make this a multidisciplinary approach.

Through the medical history and physical examination, an experienced doctor should be able to ascertain whether the female patient is suffering from any components of the triad. The existence of one triad disorder in a female athlete should be a red flag to the doctor to determine whether the other two are also present. The most important aspect of medical treatment for a female athlete with the triad of disorders is follow-up.

To break the cycle of eating disorders, which may include bingeing and purging behaviors (eating large meals, then, after feelings of guilt and shame set in, using laxatives, diuretics, or self-induced vomiting to void them from the body), experts recommend that athletes stop restricting their diets and start eating frequent, small, low-fat meals that are rich in complex carbohydrates. Small meals eaten often will quell hunger pangs, provide fuel and fluid for exercise, and increase the metabolic rate.

If the athlete is incapable of doing this, she should seek nutritional counseling.

Despite recent concerns about the female athlete triad, the benefits of regular exercise clearly outweigh the potential risks. Indeed, running offers women the same benefits as men in terms of preserving health, reducing illnesses in later life, and enhancing life at all stages by providing a regular exercise outlet.

For women seeking to avoid problems associated with menstrual irregularity, sports nutritionist Nancy Clark, author of *The Athlete's Kitchen*, (1981), and *Nancy Clark's Sports Nutrition Guidebook*, (1996) suggests the following guidelines:

• The solution may be to simply cut back on exercise by between 5 and 15 percent and eat a little more. Athletes who stop training altogether, as they may when injured, often resume their periods within two months. Some amenorrheic athletes resume their periods just by reducing exercise and experience no weight gain or a gain of less than five pounds. This small amount of weight gain may be crucial in achieving better health.

• Rather than striving to achieve an artificially low weight through excessive dieting or overexercising, female athletes should let their bodies have a greater say in determining a more natural weight. To determine appropriate weight, the female athlete should look at things such as her weight history (highest, lowest, "normal" weight), percentage of body fat, physiques of family members, and the weight at which she feels good and can comfortably remain without constant dieting. Her physician or dietitian can also provide her with unbiased professional advice.

- Do not crash diet. If she has weight to lose, the female athlete should moderately cut back on food intake by 20 percent. Severe dieters commonly stop menstruating. By following a healthy weight-reduction program, female athletes will not only have greater success with long-term weight loss, but will also have enough energy for their exercise.

- When she reaches an appropriate weight, the female athlete should practice a simple rule for eating: Eat when hungry, stop when content. If hungry all the time and obsessed with food, chances are the athlete is eating too few calories. The athlete should remember to eat enough calories to support her exercise program. As evidence suggests that amenorrhea may in part be caused by irregular eating habits (eating little at breakfast and lunch, then overeating at night; restricting diet Monday to Thursday, then gorging on weekends), female athletes should try to consume calories on a regular schedule of wholesome, well-balanced meals.

- Eat adequate protein. Research suggests that amenorrheic athletes tend to eat less protein than their regularly menstruating counterparts. It is unclear why meat seems to have a protective effect on women's periods. Nutritionists have theorized it may be that women who eat meat eat fewer calories from fiber-rich foods, and high fiber can affect hormones and calcium absorption.

A safe intake of protein for female athletes is about .5 to .75 grams per pound of body weight, which is higher than the current RDA for sedentary women. For a 120-pound woman, this is 60 to 90 grams of protein (13 to 20 percent of a 1,800 calorie diet) and is the equivalent of three or four 8-ounce servings of low-fat milk or yogurt and one 4- to 6-ounce serving of meat.

- Include small portions of red meat two or three times per week. Surveys of runners show that those with amenorrhea tend to eat less red meat than their regularly menstruating counterparts. Even though red meats can have a higher fat content than chicken or fish, an overall low-fat sports diet can accommodate some fat.

- Eat at least 20 percent of calories from fat. Amenorrheic athletes often avoid meat because they are afraid of eating fat. Some have an exaggerated perception that if they eat fat, they will get fat. Although excess calories from fat are fattening, some fat (20 to 30 percent of total calories) is an appropriate part of a healthy sports diet. Athletes can eat between 40 and 60 grams of fat a day, allowing them to balance out their diet with such foods as beef, peanut butter, cheese, and nuts.

• Eat a calcium-rich diet to help maintain bone density. Because women build peak bone density in their early adult years (twenties to thirties), the goal should be to protect against future problems of osteoporosis by eating calcium-rich foods today. A safe target is 800 to 1,200 milligrams of calcium a day. This is the equivalent of three to four servings of low-fat milk, yogurt, or other dairy or calcium-rich foods.

If the athlete is eating a very high-fiber diet (i.e., lots of bran cereal, fruits, and vegetables), there may be a greater need for calcium because the fiber may interfere with calcium absorption. For more information on preventing osteoporosis, see pages 201-204.

• Finally, Nancy Clark urges female athletes to remember that food is *health*, not just fattening calories.

For female athletes who are interested in losing weight, the following guidelines should help to do this safely and effectively:

- With a nutritionist, establish a reasonable weight goal and a realistic amount of time in which to achieve it. Do not attempt weight loss during the sport season (this may result in a loss of lean body mass). During the off-season, athletes should try to lose no more than one pound per week.
- Eat a diet that meets maximum performance needs: 60 to 70 percent complex carbohydrates, 15 to 20 percent protein, and 15 to 20 percent fat.
- Learn about proper nutrition and weight-loss strategies.
- Eliminate empty calories: foods containing simple sugars, hidden fats, and alcohol. This usually means avoiding sweet snacks and switching to healthy snacks like carrots and fruit.
- Join a weight-management group, ideally one composed chiefly of exercisers. Be sure the group includes discussion of food fads, behavioral techniques, and stress management.

Running Smart

The following safety tips for female runners are from the Road Runners Club of America (RRCA):

- Carry identification or write your name, phone number, and blood type on the inside sole of your running shoe. Include medical information.

(continued)

- Do not wear jewelry.
- Carry change for telephone calls.
- Run with a partner.
- Write down or leave word if you're running alone. Inform your friends and family of your favorite routes.
- Run in familiar areas. In unfamiliar areas contact a local RRCA club or running store.
- Know the location of telephones and open businesses and stores. Alter your route pattern.
- Always stay alert. The more aware you are, the less vulnerable you are.
- Avoid unpopulated areas, deserted streets, and overgrown trails. Especially avoid unlit areas at night. Run clear of parked cars and bushes.
- Do not wear headphones. Use your hearing to be aware of your surroundings.
- Ignore verbal harassment. Use discretion in acknowledging strangers. Look directly at others and be observant, but keep your distance and keep moving.
- Run against traffic so you can observe approaching automobiles.
- Wear reflective material if you must run before dawn or after dark.
- Use your intuition about suspicious persons or areas. Act on your intuition and avoid the person or area if you feel unsafe.
- Carry a whistle or other noisemaker.
- Call the police immediately if something happens to you or someone else, or if you notice anyone out of the ordinary during your run.

Osteoporosis

Osteoporosis is a disease that causes the bones to thin and weaken. It is one of the most common and disabling bone diseases. Though osteoporosis can affect men, it is much more likely to affect women, especially after menopause when they stop producing estrogen. Osteoporosis affects 25 percent of all postmenopausal women, or as many as 15 to 20 million American women.

A woman can prevent osteoporosis most effectively when she is in her twenties, during postpuberty bone consolidation and her attainment of peak bone mass.

Although exercise has been promoted heavily as the principal force in osteoporosis prevention, it is only one of three elements involved in preventing osteoporosis. Women also have to be sure they consume sufficient calcium and preserve their normal estrogen status (either by menstruating regularly or through estrogen replacement therapy). Although research has not yet determined the best combination of these elements, clearly all three are needed to prevent the rapid bone loss that can occur in postmenopausal women. Studies show that osteoporosis is prevalent because (1) only 22 percent of American adults do light to moderate exercise five or more times a week, (2) women are afraid of estrogen replacement therapy because media publicity has convinced them that ERT causes cancer, and (3) over 75 percent do not consume enough calcium.

Prevention Through Exercise

One of the most important means of preventing osteoporosis is regular weightbearing exercise such as running. About 30 minutes of aerobic weightbearing exercise three or four times a week is helpful for osteoporosis prevention. In addition, experts recommend that women also do strength training to stimulate the bone remodeling cycle.

However, experts unanimously caution female athletes not to rely exclusively on exercise for osteoporosis prevention. Women should exercise in conjunction with consuming high-calcium diets, maintaining estrogen status, and using proper posture.

Estrogen Status

Estrogen deficiency can cause osteoporosis. The most common cause of irregular menstruation in premenopausal women is estrogen deficiency. The athlete with exercise-induced menstrual irregularities may have bone mineral density lower than women who are menstruating regularly. For this reason, these women should seek nutritional counseling to return to menstrual regularity. This is usually done using a combination of exercise reduction and weight gain.

If a female runner fails to resume menstruating after 3 to 6 months, she should see her gynecologist. Estrogen/progesterone supplements may be prescribed. Either oral contraceptives ("the pill") or the drug Premarin-Provera can be effective in preventing further bone loss.

Calcium Intake

Inadequate calcium intake among premenopausal women is another reason women may develop osteoporosis in later life. Girls should consume 1,200 to 1,500 milligrams of calcium per day, menstruating women 1,000 milligrams per day, and nonmenstruating women 1,500 milligrams per day. However, the average American woman consumes only 400 to 600 milligrams of calcium per day. Ideally, adequate calcium intake should be achieved through a balanced diet. One dairy serving (eight ounces of milk or yogurt, one ounce of cheese) contains about 300 milligrams of calcium. Other rich sources of calcium include fish canned with bones (sardines and salmon), tofu, and green vegetables such as broccoli and snap peas.

If a female runner decides to use calcium supplements, calcium carbonate (40 percent elemental calcium) is the most concentrated form.

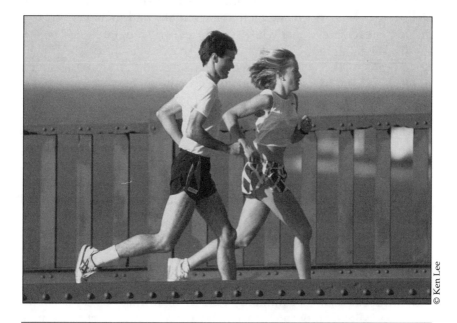

Diet and exercise play a role in the onset of premature osteoporosis and stress fractures in women.

Antacid tablets such as Tums Ex are one of the least expensive forms of calcium supplements (at 4 cents a tablet) and passed the *Consumer Reports* testing. Calcium supplements will not by themselves prevent osteoporosis but will help preserve neutral calcium balance.

Other Risk Factors

Some other risk factors predisposing women to osteoporosis include family history of osteoporosis, low body weight, cigarette smoking, race (Caucasian and Asian women are more susceptible to the disease), and lack of vitamin D.

Anemia

Part of women's lesser aerobic capacity is due to lesser amounts of hemoglobin (the iron-containing protein present in red blood cells) per blood volume as well as lesser total blood volumes. This leaves them more vulnerable to developing anemia than male athletes.

Anemia and iron deficiency are more common in female runners because of a combination of factors, including blood loss during menstruation, iron loss in sweat, inadequate dietary intake, and adolescent growth spurts. The female runner who experiences early fatigue should have a medical evaluation to check for anemia. An expert in the field is preferable because of the well-known existence of a condition known as sports anemia—a pseudo-anemia frequently seen in female runners—that is associated with increased blood volume (no specific medical care can be provided for this condition).

Iron deficiency anemia and other nutritionally related anemias are common; this merely emphasizes the need for female athletes to pay special attention to proper nutrition. Iron supplements may be necessary for those women whose diets do not contain adequate amounts of iron-rich foods such as liver, oysters, beef, turkey, dried apricots, and prune juice.

Pelvic Infection

Pelvic infections, most commonly vaginal and urinary tract infections, may occur slightly more often in female runners than in inactive women. Symptoms of vaginitis include a pus-colored, odorous discharge. The slightly higher incidence of vaginal infections can probably be explained by the accentuation of the same factors that predispose all women to infections of this kind—prolonged exposure to wet shorts and underwear, increased warmth and sweat in the area, and frictional irritation. Urinary tract infections, particularly of the bladder, are seen more often in women than men. To minimize the risks of infection, female runners should drink plenty of fluids, especially water, which increases urine flow, promoting bacterial "washout."

Contraception

Female runners use the same kinds of contraception as nonrunners. The barrier and chemical methods should have no effect on a running program, nor will their effectiveness be compromised. Occasionally, female runners develop vulvar infections caused by contraceptive cream and jelly, but this generally clears up when use is discontinued.

IUDs (intrauterine contraceptives), on the other hand, can profoundly affect female runners. They have been associated with a high incidence of pelvic pain and abnormal bleeding. The pain may persist, and during episodes, running may be impossible. IUDs are also associated with pelvic infections.

The most significant effect of IUDs on runners, however, is their potential to cause heavy, prolonged, or frequent bleeding. Some studies have shown that 75 percent of users report abnormal menstrual flow; in a third of that number, blood flow increases to the point where it requires medical attention. For runners, this blood loss can lower hemoglobin levels and therefore affect oxygen-carrying capacity. Any reduction in oxygen availability will affect training and performance.

Oral contraception ("the pill") causes many physiological changes in women. Few studies have been done, however, to determine the effect of the pill on exercise or the effect of exercise on the pill. However, it is known that changes take place. Changes that affect runners are increased blood volume and cardiac output. This suggests that the pill may actually benefit performance, although to such a minor degree as to be insignificant. Considering the research available, there is no reason to prohibit or encourage the use of the pill in female runners.

Pregnancy and Postpartum

The adaptations a healthy woman's body makes during pregnancy permit ongoing fitness participation. Not only is the risk extremely low, but exercise is beneficial for both mother and child. Common sense, proper precautions, and the advice of her obstetrician are key components in any exercise program during pregnancy.

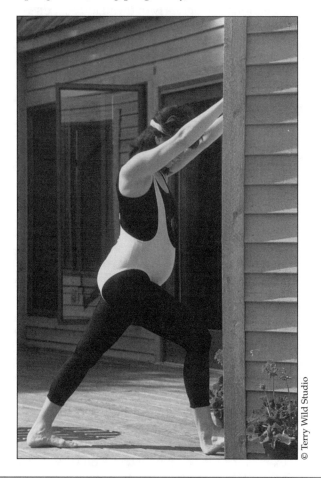

Exercise during pregnancy can be beneficial for mother and child; however, common sense and proper precautions should be a part of the exercise program.

Pregnant women should follow these general guidelines:

- Do not suddenly increase the amount of exercise undertaken nor exceed the amount performed before pregnancy.
- Eliminate sports with a high risk of injury, such as water skiing.
- Late in pregnancy, avoid excessive aerobic exercise, including long-distance running.
- Avoid exercises that require lying on the back, or those activities where balance is important.

- In the latter part of pregnancy, avoid activities likely to cause joint strains.
- Wear good supportive footwear and adequate breast support while exercising.
- Do not exercise to the point of exhaustion or severe breathlessness, and monitor pulse rate and keep within the recommended target zone.

Women should not exercise vigorously during pregnancy when there is risk of premature labor, when there is vaginal bleeding, or when placenta previa anemia, cardiac disease, thyroid disease, or hypertension is present. Exercise is not recommended when there is evidence of intrauterine growth regarding malrepresentation in the third trimester or when the woman is underweight or obese.

In many cases, pregnant women choose to suspend their outdoor running regimen because of the associated discomfort, inconvenience, and possible danger (such as from tripping, or being hit by errant cyclists or in-line skaters). Even so, many of these women will want to continue doing exercise of some kind. Pregnancy can be a time when female runners experiment with forms of aerobic exercise other than running. These exercise forms may include stationary biking, stairclimbing machines, cross-country skiing simulators, rowing machines, and aerobic dance (low-impact aerobic dance is usually more comfortable, especially in the late stages of the pregnancy). Remember that any new exercise program begun during pregnancy should be no more strenuous than the prepregnancy running program, and should be done within appropriate limitations. Most importantly, pregnant women should avoid extremes of intensity and exertion.

Also, expectant mothers should avoid sports in which there is the risk of direct trauma, such as ice-skating, outdoor biking, horseback riding, downhill skiing, and the like.

Video Exercise Programs for Pregnancy and Postpartum

The American College of Obstetricians and Gynecologists has prepared three exercise programs for pregnant women.

Pregnancy Exercise Program leads expecting women in safe exercises that can be done at home, including a warm-up routine, mild-intensity aerobic-type exercises, a cool-down routine, and a relaxation segment.

(continued)

Childbirth Preparation Program offers practice on techniques that promote relaxation and relieve discomfort during labor and childbirth. *Postnatal Exercise Program* is similar to *Pregnancy Exercise Program* but is more vigorous and aimed at toning abdominal and hip muscles and strengthening the back, yet allowing for the physical changes that persist after delivery.

The price of the video programs are $19.95 each plus $4.95 shipping and handling per order. An instruction booklet is provided with each program.

The programs are available from Healthpoints, PO Box 407, Bridgewater, Virginia 22812. They can also be ordered by calling 800-428-4488.

Pregnant women who exercise have greater nutritional requirements than those who are inactive. They must be sure to obtain enough calories to provide energy for themselves, their pregnancy, and their activity level. Pregnant women should consume an additional 30 grams of protein per day, along with the RDA of 44 grams per day for nonpregnant women. Iron from the mother's diet or from the existing stores in the body is insufficient to supply the amounts needed during pregnancy. Pregnant women should take 30 to 40 grams per day to meet the needs of their pregnancies and to maintain the woman's always-borderline iron reserves. Vitamin needs are also higher during pregnancy. Sedentary pregnant women should drink at least two quarts of fluid each day. Active pregnant women must consume more.

The goal of pregnant women who exercise should be to maintain physical fitness within the physiological limitations of pregnancy and to avoid strain or fatigue. Periods of rest and relaxation should be interspersed with the exercise. Above all, recommendations for exercise in pregnancy should be individualized.

Exercise during the portpartum period provides both physiological and psychological benefits to women runners. Many top female athletes—including champion runners—have achieved their best performance levels in the years after childbirth. As a guideline, women can resume a sports activity such as swimming or cycling within two weeks of an uncomplicated postpartum recovery. Incremental training should follow the guidelines of the American College of Obstetricians and Gynecologists, which encourage setting conservative targets to improve conditioning without risking injury. Women who are lactating have increased requirements for basic vitamins and nutrients during breast-feeding. Exercise should be structured to take into account these additional nutritional needs and should be within comfortable limits to avoid overexertion or constant fatigue.

Nutrition
for Runners

Although runners may require more food than their sedentary counterparts, in almost every other respect their nutritional requirements are identical to those of the average person. Yet nowhere else in society is there more nutritional faddism or quackery than in the sports world, and particularly in endurance sports such as running.

Athletes' obsession with diet and its effect on performance has deep historical roots. It no doubt predates organized running. Dietary superstitions of cave dwellers were predicated on the notion that eating the meat of wild animals endowed them with the qualities of those creatures—strength, endurance, and courage, for instance. In 520 BC, Greek runners switched to an all-meat diet when Eurymenes of Samos conjectured that if animals ran fast, so would humans who ate their flesh. One particularly enthusiastic disciple of this theory, Milo of Croton, is reputed to have eaten up to 20 pounds of animal flesh a day. Today the obsession is no less pronounced, and many runners, in their quest to improve performance, ingest substances as wide-ranging as glucose and dextrose, honey, gelatin, lecithin, wheat germ oil, yeast powder, phosphates, and megadoses of vitamins.

As top sports nutritionist Nancy Clark points out, the runner's diet should be designed to fuel the muscles to achieve top performance, nourish the body, and contribute to current health and nutritional longevity. And ultimately, this can be achieved not through any magic potion or pill, but through the same high-carbohydrate, low-protein diet that should be consumed by all healthy people.

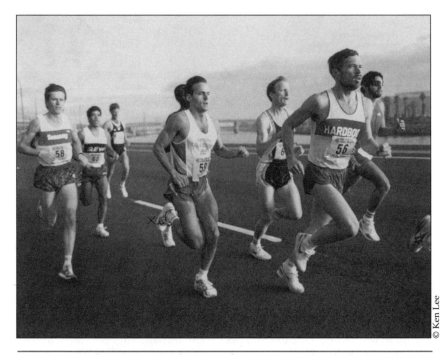

Proper nutrition fuels the muscles for top performance, nourishes the body, and contributes to overall health and longevity.

Before looking at the specific relationship between nutrition and running, general nutritional habits and some general dietary principles should be considered.

Changing Nutritional Habits

Many of us tend to eat poorly. We consume too much meat, saturated fat, cholesterol, sugar, and salt, and not enough fruit, grain (especially whole-grain products), and vegetables. These poor dietary habits, common to many Americans, are not simply a matter of overeating: calorie consumption has actually decreased during the past century. It is the types of foods being consumed that are changing.

Among the disturbing trends are the following:

- A shift from complex carbohydrates—bread, pasta, potatoes, beans, fresh fruit, and vegetables—to far less nourishing sugar
- A 30 percent increase in fat consumption since 1910

- A decline in consumption of fresh fruit, wheat flour, and potatoes and a corresponding rise in consumption of sugar, beef, poultry, corn syrup, soft drinks, and fast foods

Paralleling this undesirable shift in eating habits has been a decline in the daily expenditure of calories. Even when consuming as little as 2,000 calories a day, sedentary people often burn off less than they consume.

Making Sense of Nutrition Science: The Food Guide Pyramid

To help put sound nutritional habits into practice, the USDA has developed a food guidance program known as the food guide pyramid. It is a simplified, systematic way to ensure an adequate intake of calories and all essential nutrients that avoids the need to calculate exact amounts of protein, vitamins, minerals, and so on that are needed each day. It goes beyond the "basic food groups" once promoted by nutritionists and other health professionals. The food guide pyramid is based on the USDA's research on what foods Americans eat, what nutrients are in those foods, and how individuals can make the right food choices. The pyramid helps people choose what and how much to eat from each food group to get the nutrients needed while avoiding excessive calories, fat, cholesterol, sugar, sodium, and alcohol. The pyramid focuses on fat because most Americans' diets are too high in fat. Following the pyramid will help keep fat intake and saturated fat intake low. A diet low in fat reduces the chances of getting certain diseases and helps maintain a healthy weight. The pyramid helps individuals learn how to spot and control the sugars and salt in diet, and helps people choose foods with less sugar and salt.

The following information is based on material provided by the USDA's Human Nutrition Information Service.

What Is the Food Guide Pyramid?

The pyramid is an outline of what to eat each day. It is not a rigid prescription, but a general guide that lets individuals choose a healthful diet that is right for them. The pyramid calls for eating a variety of foods to get the nutrients needed and at the same time the right amount of calories to maintain a healthy weight. It also focuses on fat because most Americans' diets are too high in fat, especially saturated fat.

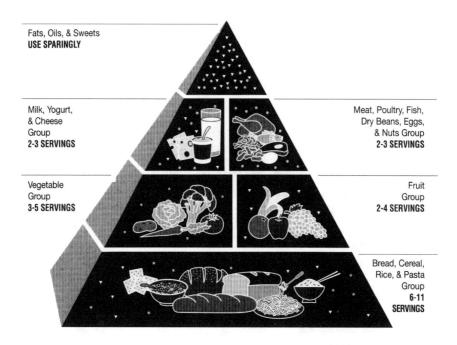

Fats, Oils, & Sweets
USE SPARINGLY

Milk, Yogurt,
& Cheese
Group
2-3 SERVINGS

Meat, Poultry, Fish,
Dry Beans, Eggs,
& Nuts Group
2-3 SERVINGS

Vegetable
Group
3-5 SERVINGS

Fruit
Group
2-4 SERVINGS

Bread, Cereal,
Rice, & Pasta
Group
**6-11
SERVINGS**

The pyramid emphasizes foods from the five major food groups shown in the lower sections of the pyramid. Each of these food groups provides some, but not all, of the nutrients needed. Foods in one group cannot replace those in another; for good health, all are needed.

A Closer Look at Fat and Added Sugars

As demonstrated in the illustration on the next page, fat and added sugars are concentrated in foods from the pyramid tip—fats, oils, and sweets. These foods supply calories, but few vitamins and minerals. By using these foods sparingly, it is possible to create a diet that supplies needed vitamins and minerals without excess calories.

Fat or sugar symbols are shown in some of the food groups because some food choices in these food groups can be high in fat and added sugars. When choosing foods for a healthful diet, consider the fat and added sugars in the food groups, as well as the fats, oils, and sweets from the pyramid tip.

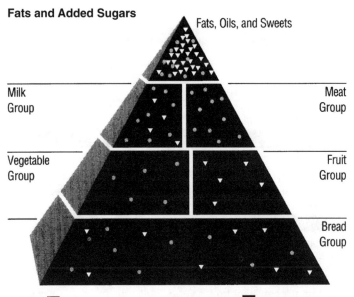

Fats and Added Sugars

Fats, Oils, and Sweets

Milk Group

Meat Group

Vegetable Group

Fruit Group

Bread Group

K E Y: ● **Fat** (naturally occurring and added) ▼ **Sugars** (added)

Fat

In general, foods that come from animals (milk and meat groups) are naturally higher in fat than foods that come from plants. But there are many low-fat dairy and lean-meat choices available, and these foods can be prepared in ways that lower fat.

Fruits, vegetables, and grain products are naturally low in fat. But many popular items are prepared with fat, like French-fried potatoes or croissants, making them higher fat choices.

For example, one baked potato has 120 calories and only minimal traces of fat, whereas 14 french fries have 225 calories and 11 grams of fat.

Added Sugars

These symbols represent sugars added to foods in processing or at the table, not the sugars found naturally in fruits and milk. It is the added sugars that provide calories with few vitamins and minerals.

Most of the added sugars in the typical American diet come from foods in the pyramid tip—soft drinks, candy, jams, jellies, syrups, and table sugar added to foods like coffee and cereal.

Added sugars in the food groups come from foods such as ice cream, sweetened yogurt, chocolate milk, canned or frozen fruit with heavy syrup, and sweetened bakery products like cakes and cookies.

Where Are the Added Sugars?

Food groups	Added sugars (teaspoons)
Bread, Cereal, Rice, and Pasta	
Bread, 1 slice	0
Doughnut, 1 medium	★★ 2
Cake, frosted, 1/16 average	★★★★★★ 6
Pie, fruit, 2 crust, 1/6 8" pie	★★★★★★ 6
Fruit	
Fruit, canned in juice, 1/2 cup	0
Fruit, canned in light syrup, 1/2 cup	★★ 2
Fruit, canned in heavy syrup, 1/2 cup	★★★★ 4
Milk, Yogurt, and Cheese	
Milk, plain, 1 cup	0
Lowfat yogurt, plain, 8 oz.	0
Lowfat yogurt, fruit, 8 oz.	★★★★★★★ 7
Ice cream, ice milk, or frozen yogurt, 1/2 cup	★★★ 3
Other	
Sugar, jam, or jelly, 1 tsp.	★ 1
Syrup or honey, 1 tbsp.	★★★ 3
Chocolate bar, 1 oz.	★★★ 3
Cola, 12 fl.oz.	★★★★★★★★★ 9
Fruit drink, ade, 12 fl.oz.	★★★★★★★★★★★★ 12

★ = 1 teaspoon sugar
Note: 4 grams of sugar = 1 teaspoon

How to Put the Pyramid Into Practice

To help you put the pyramid into practice, let's look at some common questions about how it works.

How Many Servings Are Right for Me?

The pyramid shows a range of servings for each major food group. The number of servings that are appropriate depends on how many calories the individual needs, which in turn depends on the individual's age, sex, size, and activity level. Almost everyone should have at least the minimum number of servings in the ranges.

The following calorie level suggestions are based on recommendations of the National Academy of Sciences and calorie intakes reported
by people in national food consumption surveys.

For adults and teenagers. Sixteen hundred calories is about right
for many sedentary women and some older adults. Most children, teenage girls, active women, and many sedentary men should consume
about 2,200 calories. Women who are pregnant or breast-feeding may
need somewhat more. For teenage boys, many active men, and some
very active women, 2,800 calories is about right.

For young children. It is hard to know how much food children
need to grow normally. If unsure, check with a doctor. Preschool children need the same variety of foods as older family members do, but
may need less than 1,600 calories. For fewer calories they can eat smaller
servings. However, it is important that they have the equivalent of two
cups of milk a day.

For you. Refer to the table below, which shows how many servings
are needed for a particular calorie level. For example, an active woman
who needs about 2,200 calories a day should eat nine servings of breads,
rice, or pasta. The same woman should also eat about six ounces of meat
or alternatives per day. Keep total fat (fat in the foods chosen as well as
fat used in cooking or added at the table) to about 73 grams per day.

Persons who are between calorie categories should estimate servings.

Sample Diets for a Day at 3 Calorie Levels			
	Lower (about 1,600)	Moderate (about 2,200)	Higher (about 2,800)
Bread group servings	6	9	11
Vegetable group servings	3	4	5
Fruit group servings	2	3	4
Milk group servings	2-3[1]	2-3[1]	2-3[1]
Meat group[2] (ounces)	5	6	7
Total fat (grams)	53	73	93
Total added sugars (teaspoons)	6	12	18

[1]Women who are pregnant or breast-feeding, teenagers, and young adults
to age 24 need 3 servings.
[2]Meat group amounts are in total ounces.

For example, some less active women may need only 2,000 calories to maintain a healthy weight. At that calorie level, eight servings of breads would be about right.

What Is a Serving?

The amount of food that counts as a serving is listed in the table below. Someone who eats a larger portion should count it as more than one serving. For example, a half cup of cooked pasta counts as one serving in the bread, rice, cereal, and pasta group. If a person eats one cup of pasta, that would be two servings. Conversely, a person who eats a smaller portion should count it as part of a serving.

What Counts as a Serving?

Food groups

Bread, Cereal, Rice, and Pasta

1 slice of bread	1 ounce of ready-to-eat cereal	1/2 cup of cooked cereal, rice, or pasta

Vegetable

1 cup of raw leafy vegetables	1/2 cup of other vegetables, cooked or chopped raw	3/4 cup of vegetable juice

Fruit

1 medium apple, banana, orange	1/2 cup of chopped, cooked, or canned fruit	3/4 cup of fruit juice

Milk, Yogurt, and Cheese

1 cup of milk or yogurt	1-1/2 ounces of natural cheese	2 ounces of processed cheese

Meat, Poultry, Fish, Dry Beans, Eggs, and Nuts

2-3 ounces of cooked lean meat, poultry, or fish	1/2 cup of cooked dry beans, 1 egg, or 2 tablespoons of peanut butter count as 1 ounce of lean meat

Isn't 6 to 11 Servings of Breads and Cereals a Lot?

It may sound like a lot, but it's not. For example, a slice of bread is one serving, so a sandwich for lunch would equal two servings. A small bowl of cereal and one slice of toast for breakfast are two more servings.

And a cup of rice or pasta for dinner adds two more servings. A snack of three or four small plain crackers adds yet another serving. That comes to seven servings, which proves it adds up quicker than most people think.

Do I Need to Measure Servings?

No. Use servings only as a general guide. For mixed foods, estimate the main ingredients as best you can. For example, a generous serving of pizza would count in the bread group (crust), the milk group (cheese), and the vegetable group (tomato); a helping of beef stew would count in the meat group and the vegetable group. Both have some fat—fat in the cheese on the pizza and in the gravy from the stew if it is made from meat drippings.

What if I Want to Lose or Gain Weight?

The best and simplest way to lose weight is to increase physical activity and reduce fat and sugars in the diet. Be sure to eat at least the minimum number of servings from the five major food groups in the food guide pyramid. They are needed for the vitamins, minerals, carbohydrates, and protein they provide. Try to pick the lowest fat choices from the food groups.

To gain weight, increase the amounts of foods eaten from all the food groups. Anyone who loses weight unexpectedly should see a doctor.

How Much Fat Can I Have?

It depends on individual calorie needs. The dietary guidelines recommend that Americans limit fat in their diets to 30 percent of calories. This amounts to 53 grams of fat in a 1,600-calorie diet, 73 grams of fat in a 2,200-calorie diet, and 93 grams of fat in a 2,800-calorie diet.

A person will get half this fat even when they pick the lowest fat choices from each food group and add no fat to foods in preparation or at the table.

Individuals should decide how to use the additional fat in their daily diets. Some may want to have foods from the five major food groups that are higher in fat, such as whole milk instead of skim milk. Others may want to use it in cooking or at the table in the form of spreads, dressings, or toppings.

How Do I Check My Diet for Fat?

Those who want to be sure that they have a low-fat diet should count the grams of fat in their day's food choices using the pyramid food choices chart and compare them to the number of grams of fat suggested for their calorie level.

It is not necessary to count fat grams every day, but doing a fat checkup occasionally will help keep a person on the right track. Those who discover they are eating too much fat should choose lower-fat foods more often.

Are Some Types of Fat Worse Than Others?

Yes. Eating too much saturated fat raises blood cholesterol levels in many people, increasing their risk for heart disease. The dietary guidelines recommend limiting saturated fat to less than 10 percent of calories, or about one-third of total fat intake.

All fats in food are mixtures of three types of fatty acids—saturated, monounsaturated, and polyunsaturated.

- *Saturated fats* are found in the largest amounts in fats from meat and dairy products and in some vegetable fats such as coconut, palm, and palm kernel oils.
- *Monounsaturated fats* are found mainly in olive, peanut, and canola oils.
- *Polyunsaturated fats* are found mainly in safflower, sunflower, corn, soybean, and cottonseed oils, and some fish.

How Do I Avoid Too Much Saturated Fat?

Follow the food guide pyramid, keeping total fat within recommended levels. Choose fat from a variety of food sources, but mostly from those foods higher in polyunsaturated or monounsaturated fat.

What About Cholesterol?

Cholesterol and fat are not the same thing. Cholesterol is a fatlike substance present in all animal foods—meat, poultry, fish, milk and milk products, and egg yolks. Both the lean and fat of meat and the meat and skin of poultry contain cholesterol. In milk products, cholesterol is mostly in the fat, so lower-fat products contain less cholesterol. Egg yolks and organ meats, like liver, are high in cholesterol. Plant foods do not contain cholesterol.

Dietary cholesterol, as well as saturated fat, raises blood cholesterol levels in many people, increasing their risk for heart disease. Some health authorities recommend that dietary cholesterol be limited to an average of 300 milligrams or less per day. To keep dietary cholesterol to this level, follow the food guide pyramid, keeping total fat down to the appropriate amount. It is not necessary to eliminate all foods that are high in cholesterol. Have three to four egg yolks a week, counting those used as ingredients in custards and baked products. Use lower-fat dairy products often and occasionally include dry beans and peas in place of meat.

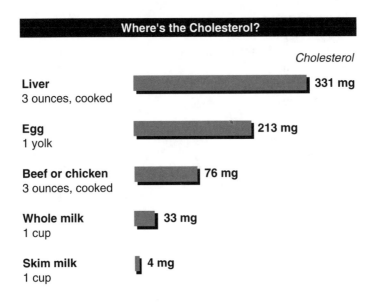

Where's the Cholesterol?

Cholesterol

Liver
3 ounces, cooked .... 331 mg

Egg
1 yolk .... 213 mg

Beef or chicken
3 ounces, cooked .... 76 mg

Whole milk
1 cup .... 33 mg

Skim milk
1 cup .... 4 mg

Cholesterol and Diet

Cholesterol is a fatty substance produced by the body and is found in foods of animal origin. Cholesterol serves many vital functions in the body, but excessive amounts in the diet may be harmful. Coronary heart disease is the most serious disease associated with high cholesterol levels.

A simple blood cholesterol test can be performed to evaluate cholesterol levels. To be in the low-risk category for developing coronary heart disease, total cholesterol should be below 200 mg/d*, LDL cholesterol below 130 mg/d, HDL cholesterol above 35 to 50 mg/d, and the ratio of total cholesterol to HDL cholesterol should be 3.0 to 4.5 or less for men and 3.0 to 4.0 or less for women.

(continued)

Cholesterol levels in average servings of food

Meat, Fish, Poultry, Eggs (average serving after cooking)	Milligrams Cholesterol
Liver (3 oz, 85 gm)	372
Egg (1 large, 50 gm)	252
Shrimp, canned, drained (3 oz, 85 gm)	128
Veal (3 oz, 85 gm)	86
Lamb (3 oz, 85 gm)	83
Beef (3 oz, 85 gm)	80
Pork (3 oz, 85 gm)	76
Chicken breast ($^1/_2$ breast, 80 gm)	63
Lobster (3 oz, 85 gm)	72
Clams, canned, drained ($^1/_2$ cup, 80 gm)	50
Chicken drumstick (1, 43 gm)	39
Oysters, canned (3 oz, 85 gm)	38
Fish, fillet (3 oz, 85 gm)	34-75

Dairy Foods (average serving)	Milligrams Cholesterol
Whole milk (8 oz, 244 gm)	34
Cheddar or Swiss cheese (1 oz, 28 gm)	28
Ice cream ($^1/_2$ cup, 67 gm)	27-49
American processed cheese (1 oz, 28 gm)	25
Low fat (2%) milk (8 oz, 246 gm)	22
Heavy whipping cream (1 tbsp, 15 gm)	20
Yogurt, plain or vanilla (1 cup, 227 gm)	17
Cream cheese (1 tbsp, 14 gm)	16
Cottage cheese ($^1/_2$ cup, 134 gm)	12-24
Butter (1 tsp, 5 gm)	12
Sour cream (1tbsp, 12 gm)	8
Half-and-half (1 tbsp, 15 gm)	6
Cottage cheese, dry curd ($^1/_2$ cup, 100 gm)	6
Skim milk and buttermilk (8 oz, 245 gm)	5

Desserts (average serving)	Milligrams Cholesterol
Lady fingers (4, 44 gm)	157
Custard ($^1/_2$ cup, 133 gm)	139
Apple pie (1/8 of 9" pie, 144 gm)	120

(continued)

Custard pie ($^1/_8$ of 9" pie, 114 gm)	120
Lemon meringue pie ($^1/_8$ of 9" pie, 105 gm)	98
Bread pudding with raisins ($^1/_2$ cup, 133 gm)	95
Peach pie ($^1/_8$ of 9" pie, 114 gm)	70
Pumpkin pie ($^1/_8$ of 9" pie, 144 gm)	70
Yellow cake, from mix ($^1/_{16}$ of 9" cake, 75 gm)	36
Chocolate cake, from mix ($^1/_{16}$ of 9" cake, 69 gm)	33
Brownie, homemade (1, 20 gm)	17
Chocolate pudding, from mix ($^1/_2$ cup, 130 gm	15
Rice pudding with raisins ($^1/_2$ cup, 133 gm)	15

*mg/d = number of mg of cholesterol per 100 cc of blood

What About Sugars?

Choosing a diet low in fat is a concern for everyone; choosing one low in sugars is also important for people who have low calorie needs. Sugars include white sugar, brown sugar, raw sugar, corn syrup, honey, and molasses; these supply calories and little else nutritionally.

To avoid getting too many calories from sugars, try to limit added sugars to 6 teaspoons a day when eating a 1,600-calorie diet, 12 teaspoons at 2,200 calories, or 18 teaspoons at 2,800 calories. These amounts are intended to be averages over time. The patterns are illustrations of healthful proportions in the diet, not rigid prescriptions.

Added sugars are in foods like candy and soft drinks, as well as in jams, jellies, and sugar added at the table. Some added sugars are also in foods from the food groups, such as chocolate milk and fruit canned in heavy syrup. See page 216 for the approximate amount of sugars in some popular foods.

Sugar Use and Abuse

The preactivity "sugar fix" is currently a subject of controversy. Athletes have long believed that eating a candy bar or drinking a can of cola immediately before their activity will give them a "sugar rush" and a boost of energy. Until recently, however, the informed

(continued)

judgment was that consuming sugar right before exercise impairs performance because the quick energy lift athletes are seeking is brought on by a rapid rise in blood glucose and a release of extra insulin. The combined effect of insulin and exercise may cause the blood sugar level to plummet, a condition known as hypoglycemia, and make the athlete feel light-headed, shaky, and uncoordinated. Gastric distress was thought to be another side effect of a sugar-intensive preexercise snack.

Recent evidence, however, suggests the sugar fix may not be so bad after all. Researchers at the University of Pennsylvania concluded that temporary hypoglycemia doesn't impair performance in high-intensity exercise. They also reported that none of the cyclists who had been given chocolate bars before a grueling race had suffered stomach problems. This study differs, however, from the landmark research done in the late 1970s by David Costill and his colleagues at the Human Performance Laboratory at Ball State University, in which the subjects were given highly concentrated glucose rather than candy bars, which contain fat and caffeine as well as sugar. The studies also differed in the length of time between ingestion and exercise and in the duration and intensity of the exercise.

What is the recreational athlete to make of the controversy? For now, most nutritionists are not changing their directives to athletes. They admit that the sugar fix provides energy, but recommend that the energy come from a more nutritious source, such as yogurt, juice, soft pretzels, bananas, or simple sandwiches. The primary consideration for recreational athletes is that relying on a sugar fix depends on insulin sensitivity and nutrition preferences.

Do I Have to Give Up Salt?

No. But most people eat more than they need. Some health authorities say that sodium intake should be no more than 3,000 milligrams a day; some say no more than 2,400 milligrams. Much of the sodium people consume comes from salt they add while cooking and at the table (one teaspoon of salt provides about 2,000 milligrams of sodium).

Go easy on salt and foods that are high in sodium, including cured meats, luncheon meats, many cheeses, most canned soups and vegetables, and soy sauce. Look for lower salt and no-salt-added versions of these products at your supermarket.

Refer to the following table for an idea of the amount of sodium in different types of foods. Information on food labels can also help consumers make food choices to keep sodium intake moderate.

Where's the Salt?

Food groups	Sodium, mg
Bread, Cereal, Rice, and Pasta	
Cooked cereal, rice, pasta, unsalted, 1/2 cup	Trace
Ready-to-eat cereal, 1 oz.	100-360
Bread, 1 slice	110-175
Vegetable	
Vegetables, fresh or frozen, cooked without salt, 1/2 cup	Less than 70
Vegetables, canned or frozen with sauce, 1/2 cup	140-460
Tomato juice, canned, 3/4 cup	660
Vegetable soup, canned, 1 cup	820
Fruit	
Fruit, fresh, frozen, canned, 1/2 cup	Trace
Milk, Yogurt, and Cheese	
Milk, 1 cup	120
Yogurt, 8 oz.	160
Natural cheeses, 1-1/2 oz.	110-450
Processed cheeses, 2 oz.	800
Meat, Poultry, Fish, Dry Beans, Eggs, and Nuts	
Fresh meat, poultry, fish, 3 oz.	Less than 90
Tuna, canned, water pack, 3 oz.	300
Bologna, 2 oz.	580
Ham, lean, roasted, 3 oz.	1,020
Other	
Salad dressing, 1 tbsp.	75-220
Ketchup, mustard, steak sauce, 1 tbsp.	130-230
Soy sauce, 1 tbsp.	1,030
Salt, 1 tsp.	2,000
Dill pickle, 1 medium	930
Potato chips, salted, 1 oz.	130
Corn chips, salted, 1 oz.	235
Peanuts, roasted in oil, salted, 1 oz.	120

A Closer Look at the Food Groups

To help runners make good nutritional food choices, we take a quick look at the importance of each of the food groups and give selection tips (see page 218 for serving measurements for each group).

Breads, Cereals, Rice, and Pasta

These foods provide complex carbohydrates (starches), which are a rich source of energy, especially in low-fat diets. They also provide vitamins, minerals, and fiber. The food guide pyramid suggests 6 to 11 servings of these foods a day.

Aren't starchy foods fattening? No. It is what is added to these foods or cooked with them that adds most of the calories. For example, margarine or butter on bread, cream or cheese sauces on pasta, and the sugar and fat used with flour in making cookies add most of the calories to these foods.

Selection tips:

- To get enough fiber, choose several servings a day of foods made from whole grains, such as whole wheat bread and whole grain cereals.
- Choose most often foods that contain little fat or sugars. These include bread, English muffins, rice, and pasta.
- Baked goods made from flour, such as cakes, cookies, croissants, and pastries, count as part of this food group, but they are high in fat and sugars.
- Be conservative when adding spreads, seasonings, or toppings, as these contain large amounts of fat and sugars.
- When preparing pasta, stuffing, and sauce from the packaged mixes, use only half the butter or margarine; if milk or cream is called for, use low-fat milk.

Vegetables

Vegetables provide vitamins, such as A and C and folate, and minerals such as iron and magnesium. They are naturally low in fat and provide fiber. The food guide pyramid suggests three to five servings of these foods a day.

Selection tips:

- Different types of vegetables provide different nutrients. For variety eat

  — dark green leafy vegetables (spinach, romaine lettuce, broccoli),
  — deep yellow vegetables (carrots, sweet potatoes),
  — starchy vegetables (potatoes, corn, peas),
  — legumes (navy, pinto, and kidney beans, chickpeas), and
  — other vegetables (lettuce, tomatoes, onions, green beans).

- Include dark green leafy vegetables and legumes several times a week—they are especially good sources of vitamins and minerals. Legumes also provide protein and can be used in place of meat.
- Be conservative with fat added to vegetables at the table or during cooking. Added spreads such as butter, mayonnaise, and salad dressing count as fat.
- Use low-fat salad dressing.

Fruits

Fruits and fruit juices provide important amounts of vitamins A and C and potassium. They are low in fat and sodium. The food guide pyramid suggests two to four servings of fruits a day.

Selection tips:

- Choose fresh fruits, fruit juices, and frozen, canned, or dried fruit. Pass up fruit canned or frozen in heavy syrups and sweetened fruit juices.
- Eat whole fruits often; they are higher in fiber than fruit juices.
- Have citrus fruits, melons, and berries regularly. They are rich in vitamin C.
- Count only 100 percent fruit juice as fruit. Punches, ades, and most fruit "drinks" contain only a little juice and lots of added sugars. Grape and orange sodas do not count as fruit juice.

Meat, Poultry, Fish, Dry Beans, Eggs, and Nuts

Meat, poultry, and fish supply protein, B vitamins, iron, and zinc. The other foods in this group—dry beans, eggs, and nuts—are similar to meats in providing protein and most vitamins and minerals. The food guide pyramid suggests two to three servings each day of foods from this group. The total amount of these servings should be the equivalent of five to seven ounces of cooked lean meat, poultry, or fish per day.

Selection tips:

- Choose lean meats, poultry without skin, fish, and dry beans and peas often. They are the choices lowest in fat.
- Prepare meats in low-fat ways:
    — Trim away as much of the fat as possible.
    — Broil, roast, or boil these foods instead of frying them.
- Eat egg yolks sparingly; they are high in cholesterol. Use only one yolk per person in egg dishes. Make larger portions by adding extra egg whites.
- Nuts and seeds are high in fat, so eat them in moderation.

Milk, Yogurt, and Cheese

Milk products provide protein, vitamins, and minerals. Milk, yogurt, and cheese are the best sources of calcium. The food guide pyramid suggests two to three servings of milk, yogurt, and cheese a day—two for most people, and three for women who are pregnant or breast-feeding, teenagers, and young adults to age 24.

Selection tips:

- Choose skim milk and nonfat yogurt often. They are lowest in fat.
- One and a half to two ounces of cheese and eight ounces of yogurt count as a serving from this group because they supply the same amount of calcium as one cup of milk.
- Cottage cheese is lower in calcium than most cheeses. One cup of cottage cheese counts as only a half serving of milk.
- Eat high-fat cheese and ice cream sparingly. They can add much fat (especially saturated fat) to a diet.
- Choose part skim or low-fat cheeses when available and lower-fat milk desserts, like ice milk or frozen yogurt.

Running Nutrition Basics

Runners perform best on a high-carbohydrate, low-protein diet. A wholesome diet based on carbohydrates (between 55 and 65 percent of daily caloric intake) including meat or protein-rich foods as the accompaniment (10 to 15 percent of caloric intake) and fat for the remaining calories (about 25 to 30 percent of caloric intake) is appropriate for all athletes. This diet should include foods from all the main food groups (at least 6 to 11 servings of breads, cereals, rice, and pastas; 3 to 5 servings of vegetables; 2 to 4 servings of fruit; 2 to 3 servings from the meat, poultry, fish, dry beans, eggs, and nuts group; and 2 to 3 servings from the milk, yogurt, and cheese group) that not only taste good, but are high in nutrients and are easy to digest.

Carbohydrates

Carbohydrates are the most important energy source during intense physical activity. Carbs, as they are colloquially known, come in two forms: simple and complex. Simple carbohydrates are found in fruits, juices, milk, frozen yogurt, and candy, while complex carbohydrates are found in whole grains, vegetables, pasta, rice, and breads. The body breaks down both forms of carbohydrates into glucose for immediate energy needs. Excess glucose is stored mainly in the muscles, and to a lesser degree in the liver, as glycogen to fuel exercise. While it is the most important nutrient, carbohydrate is also the least abundant nutrient stored in the body. Just two hours of exercise or eight hours of fasting can significantly deplete carbohydrate stores. In runners, depleted glycogen stores can cause fatigue and poor performance.

Sport nutritionists generally recommend a carbohydrate intake of about three to four grams of carbohydrates per pound of body weight per day, or a minimum of 500 grams of carbohydrates per day, particularly for endurance athletes such as runners. For example, a 180-pound athlete would need about 700 grams of carbohydrates (2,800 calories) per day. This means eating a great deal of pasta and vegetables: one baked potato is about 21 grams of carbohydrates, an apple about 18 grams, and a bowl of Cheerios about 20 grams.

Besides consuming a high-carbohydrate diet as part of a daily health regimen, a runner should consume carbohydrates soon after training to maximize recovery.

Carbo Loading for the Big Event

Many endurance athletes use carbohydrate-loading programs prior to competition.

The body converts carbohydrates into blood glucose and glycogen. The latter is a form of carbohydrate that is stored in the muscles

(continued)

and liver in limited amounts. During exercise, the body draws on its glycogen stores for fuel; if the exercise is demanding, total glycogen reserves can be used up after two hours. If the reserves are not sufficient to begin with, the result is early fatigue. The key to increasing performance in endurance events through nutrition is to begin competition with maximum levels of glycogen in the muscles, which allows athletes to perform at a higher pace for longer periods.

Traditional method

The classic method of carbohydrate loading, first developed by Scandinavian researchers a quarter century ago, involves severely depleting the glycogen stores through exercise a week or so before a major competition, and then drastically reducing carbohydrate intake for the next several days. Three days prior to competition, the athlete dramatically reduces or cuts out training and increases carbohydrate intake to the point where it represents up to 90 percent of calorie intake. The glycogen-starved muscles absorb the carbohydrates in an extremely concentrated form and thus increase their endurance. Unfortunately, there are numerous undesirable side effects associated with the depletion phase of the traditional carbo-loading regimen, including dizziness, muscle soreness, irritability, and fatigue, which has prompted less extreme methods of increasing glycogen stores in the body.

Updated method

An updated carbohydrate-loading technique eliminates many of the problems associated with the traditional method and is more appropriate for the recreational athlete. In this updated method, the athlete eats a normal mixed diet (about 50 percent of calories from carbohydrates) instead of the low-carbohydrate diet of the traditional regimen. Training is reduced during this period. Then, for the following three days, the athlete eats a high-carbohydrate diet (70 percent of calories from carbohydrates). This updated technique of carbohydrate loading creates glycogen stores equal to those of the traditional method.

In this shortened version of the carbohydrate-loading regimen, the athlete eats a high-carbohydrate diet for the three days prior

(continued)

to the event, trains moderately for the first two days, and rests on the day immediately preceding the event.

Consumption of carbohydrates should be increased from a normal 350 grams to 550 to 600 grams. Any consumption in excess of 600 grams will not result in greater concentrations of glycogen in the muscles, and the excess will probably be converted into fat.

Choice of carbohydrates

The athlete should choose complex carbohydrates, as these provide higher concentrations of glycogen than do simple carbohydrates such as candy. When most athletes think of carbohydrates, they automatically think of pasta products, not realizing that carbohydrates are concentrated in fruit and are the primary nutrient in most vegetables. Refer to table 11.1 on page 238 for a list of convenient carbohydrate-rich foods and their specific carbohydrate contents.

Protein

Protein is necessary to build and repair muscle, ligaments, tendons, and other tissue. It is not a particularly useful energy source. Less than 10 percent of the energy used during training comes from protein breakdown. Runners need only about one-half to one gram of protein per pound of body weight per day. Only a limited amount of protein is needed for tissue building. Excess protein is turned into fat.

If the total intake of carbohydrates is insufficient, the body turns to protein to produce energy instead of using it to do its intended job—tissue building. In such cases, the body starts losing lean muscle mass.

A small serving of protein-rich food (lean meat, poultry, seafood, dairy products, and beans) at each meal is enough to support a strenuous schedule and fulfill the body's basic requirements. Protein supplements are not necessary for runners who are meeting their overall daily caloric needs.

Fat

Fats, the most concentrated energy source of the dietary nutrients, are classified as either saturated or unsaturated (polyunsaturated or monounsaturated). Saturated fatty acids (fat in beef, pork, lamb and poultry, dairy products, coconut oil, palm oil, hydrogenated oil, and chocolate) tend to increase blood cholesterol levels. Saturated fats should provide no more than 10 percent of the daily caloric intake. Polyunsaturated fats come primarily from vegetable oils (corn, cottonseed, safflower, soybean, and sunflower oils) and from fish oils. Monounsaturated fats are found in avocados, canola oil, olive oil, peanut oil, and most nuts.

Most Americans have plenty of fat, and need to consume only minimal amounts to provide calorie intake. The average person has sufficient fat energy available to run 1,000 miles (but would run out of carbohydrates in 15 to 20 miles). Besides providing energy, fat provides insulation and shock protection, transports certain vitamins through the sys-

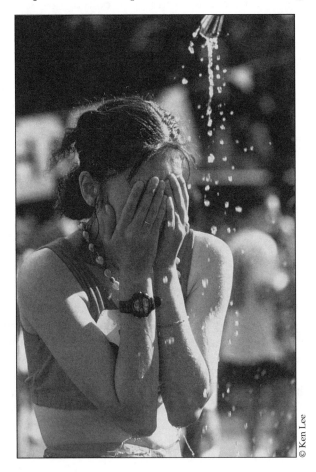

© Ken Lee

Just two hours of running can significantly decrease carbohydrate stores; however, the average person has sufficient fat energy available to run 1,000 miles.

tem, and supplies essential fatty acids. Dietary fats should provide 10 to 30 percent of daily caloric intake—a major reduction in the typical American diet. Despite increased awareness of the health risks associated with a high-fat diet, consuming too little fat creates other problems for the athlete, in particular inadequate calorie intake. Some fat at each meal is appropriate, but avoid excessive amounts of fried, greasy, oily, and buttery foods, which will fill the stomach but leave the muscles unfueled.

Vitamins and Minerals

Vitamins and minerals are important for a variety of metabolic reactions, but they provide no energy. There is a widespread misconception among runners that vitamin supplements will enhance athletic performance.

Many runners consume large quantities of vitamin-mineral supplements in the belief that these dosages will improve performance. Medical science, however, offers no evidence that performance is improved by consumption of these supplements. The American Medical Association states that healthy men or women who aren't pregnant or breastfeeding do not require vitamin-mineral supplements so long as they are eating a varied diet.

The AMA's most recent report on the subject conceded that, due to the changing dietary habits of Americans (increased consumption of processed foods and meals on the run), there may be many people whose vitamin-mineral intake is insufficient. Before resorting to supplements, however, these individuals should improve their diets.

When runners use a supplement, the dose should never exceed 150 percent of the recommended dietary allowance (RDA). Although most nutritionists agree that no harm will come of taking this amount, they also state that there is no evidence this practice is helpful.

The AMA report states that supplements containing 2 to 10 times the RDA of any vitamin should be taken only under medical supervision when an individual has a specific disease for which the vitamins are prescribed.

Taking megadoses of vitamins—an increasingly popular tactic among runners—is condemned by the AMA. Megadose therapy is costly and builds false hopes. Of greater concern to medical professionals is evidence that massive consumption of vitamins and minerals can be toxic and can impair the delicate metabolic relationships between vital nutrients.

The truth is this: Supplements of vitamins or minerals exceeding the RDA will not improve the performance of well-nourished athletes.

Fluids

Runners should emphasize fluids as part of a healthy diet. Proper hydration is the most frequently overlooked aid to athletic performance.

Fluids are necessary to regulate body temperature and prevent overheating. For example, if a runner loses three to four pounds during practice or training, he or she will be less able to reduce body heat. This failure to regulate temperature will drastically hurt performance and can cause medical problems. Besides regulating temperature, fluids also transport energy, vitamins, and minerals throughout the circulatory system. Everyone should drink at least six to eight glasses of water daily or until the urine is a clear color. Runners should also drink copious amounts of fluid before, during, and after exercise. Frequent urination is a positive sign that enough fluids are being consumed. A simple way to determine how much fluid to drink is to be weighed before and after a workout or competition. The weight loss will be almost entirely fluids and the runner should replace it accordingly (one pound of lost sweat equals two cups of fluid). Drinking *more* fluid rather than less can help prevent dehydration and overheating. Fluids can include water, juices, or sports drinks.

Fluid Replacement: Sports Drinks Versus Water

Drinking fluids while exercising is crucial for sports performance. But what fluids should the athlete drink? In addition to water, athletes can choose from a variety of sports drinks, including Gatorade, Recharge, and Vitalade.

For casual athletes, water is sufficient for fluid replacement. If the exercise lasts longer than 30 minutes (especially in high temperature or humidity), the participant should drink a cup of cool water every 15 to 20 minutes. Athletes shouldn't wait until they are thirsty before drinking, as the thirst drive lags behind actual needs. A drop in body weight of 2 to 4 percent will affect performance. For example, 10K race times may be slowed by 4 to 8 percent. Weight losses of more than 4 percent can raise temperature and cause heat cramps, heat illness, heat stroke, and even death.

For endurance activities lasting longer than two hours, sports performance doesn't depend just on water balance, but on blood sugar levels, too. In these cases, many sports drinks provide water

(continued)

in a readily absorbed solution and supply a small amount of sugar and sodium. Current research suggests that athletes in endurance sports benefit more from sports drinks than from water. Several types of sugar (glucose, sucrose, fructose, or maltodextrin) are contained in sports drinks. All have similar properties except fructose, which may hamper water absorption and irritate the stomach if it is the prime energy source.

Some sports drinks use glucose polymers to boost the sugar content of the drink without affecting the rate of water absorption. These drinks offer approximately a 20 percent sugar solution, providing a significant amount of sugar. This can be very beneficial during ultraendurance events in which muscle and liver glycogen stores are depleted.

Several glucose polymer drinks currently available include: Exceed fluid replacement drink (Ross), Bodyfuel 450 (Vitex Foods), and Cytomax.

After exercise, rehydration occurs more quickly when the fluid used contains small amounts of sodium as compared with plain water. Sports drinks provide this small amount of sodium (50 to 200 milligrams per eight fluid ounces) for this purpose.

Meal Timing and Running Nutrition

Maintaining adequate carbohydrate stores does not just require eating properly on a daily basis. It also entails planning for meals immediately before and after exercise, and sometimes during the event itself.

Before Running

Runners should eat a light meal three to six hours before the vigorous exercise. The meal should provide 75 to 150 grams of carbohydrates to supplement glycogen stores. As protein is virtually useless as a source of immediate energy, and contributes to dehydration because it increases the need to urinate, protein should constitute a very small part of the preactivity meal. For instance, if the preactivity meal of choice is pasta, the sauce should contain little meat; if it is a sandwich, the bread should be thickly sliced and contain just a small amount of meat (preferably turkey or chicken). The meal should be low in fat since fats take longer to digest. Fat slows emptying of the stomach and upper gastrointestinal tract, thereby impairing breathing and placing increased strain on circulation, eventually leading to nausea.

Runners should choose foods that are familiar and easy to digest. Liquid meals offer convenience and rapid absorption into the system, but the runner should test them in training before using them in an important event.

As we have seen, the runner should plan prerun meals so the stomach is empty by the time he or she begins to exercise. This will prevent nausea and gastrointestinal upset. The larger the calorie content of the meal, the longer it takes to digest. Time requirements for digestion of various-sized meals are

- four to six hours for a large meal,
- two to three hours for a smaller meal (less than 500 calories),
- one to two hours for a blended or liquid meal, and
- less than an hour for a light snack (piece of fruit, small bowl of cereal).

For those who wish to run in the morning but who do not want to wake early and eat a large meal, the best choice is to eat a large carbohydrate-rich meal relatively late the night before, then a small breakfast two hours before the run.

Drinking 8 to 12 ounces of cold water 10 to 15 minutes before exercising is advisable, especially if the runner is susceptible to dehydration. Cold drinks offer the advantage of emptying more rapidly from the stomach and at the same time enhancing body cooling.

During Running

Runners should eat carbohydrates during events lasting longer than 90 minutes. Consuming these carbohydrates will improve stamina and performance. Carbohydrates also help maintain normal blood sugar levels as well as provide a source of energy for the muscles. The harder a person runs, the more likely he or she will be to require food during the run. Solid food snacks such as bananas, fig bars, and bagels can be eaten and digested during exercise and are ideal for participants in long-distance events.

As thirst is not an effective indicator of fluid needs during training and prolonged periods of exertion, runners need to force themselves to drink more. Even partial rehydration can minimize the risks of overheating and the stress on circulation. There is also a well-known psychological lift associated with consuming liquids during competition. To be readily available for rehydration and cooling, fluids must quickly leave the stomach. For this reason, how much the runner drinks, the temperature of what he or she drinks, and what type of liquid is consumed are of importance.

Although large quantities of fluid leave the stomach quickly, they can cause stomach upsets. For this reason, it is preferable to drink small volumes of fluid more frequently (three to five ounces every 15 minutes).

As discussed in the previous section, cold drinks have the advantage of leaving the stomach more quickly and at the same time encouraging body cooling. In most situations, plain water is preferred.

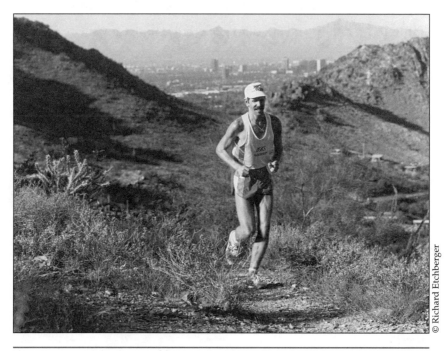

Thirst is not a good indicator of fluid needs; athletes should drink before they are thirsty.

After Running

Carbohydrate intake is also important after vigorous physical exertion. Glycogen in muscles is replaced most rapidly during the hours immediately following exercise. In the first 30 minutes after exercising, runners should consume at least 100 grams of carbohydrates, followed by a similar intake two to four hours later. This is especially important after intensive events when the runner wants to return quite soon to his or her training schedule.

In what form these carbohydrates are consumed doesn't matter. Initially, liquid carbohydrate sources such as polymer drinks may be more convenient and palatable, and may contribute to rehydration. Juices are an especially effective source of liquid carbohydrates. Fruit, pasta, or other solid carbohydrates may taste better a little later. Refer to table 11.1 for a list of the carbohydrate content (in grams) of a few liquid and solid foods.

To calculate how much fluid to drink after vigorous exercise, runners should weigh themselves before and after the activity. This may not be practical before every session, so the athlete should be familiar with approximately how much fluid weight he or she loses during exercise.

Table 11.1 Liquid and Solid Food Carbohydrate Content

Food	Amount	Carbohydrates (grams)
Fruit		
Orange	1 medium	64
Raisins	$^1/_4$ cup	30
Apricots	4	30
Banana	1	25
Apple	1 medium	20
Grapes	1 cup	16
Juice (apple/orange)	1 cup	30
Bread		
Hero roll	8"	60
Bran muffin	1	45
Pancakes	3 medium	42
Vegetables		
Baked potato	1 large	55
Baked beans	1 cup	50
Rice	1 cup	50
Corn	1 cup	31
Carrot	1 medium	7
Others		
Commercial high carbohydrate drink	12 oz	70-90
Yogurt (strawberry)	1 cup	43
Egg noodles	1 cup	37

For each pound of weight lost during exertion, the runner should drink at least two cups of fluids. Another effective way to monitor hydration is through urination; the runner is adequately hydrated if his or her urine is clear; darker yellow urine is a sign that the runner needs to consume more fluids.

Nutritional Considerations of the Female Runner

Although women's nutritional requirements are much the same as their male counterparts, there are certain important differences, notably their special needs for vitamins and nutrients such as iron, calcium, and estrogen. As mentioned in previous chapters, poor nutrition in women can have disastrous consequences when combined with a vigorous exercise regimen. Female runners, whether they be professional or recreational athletes, need to be vigilant about their nutritional intake. For a thorough discussion of how diet and exercise play a role in overuse injuries in female athletes—as well as nutritional guidelines for avoiding problems caused by menstrual irregularity—see chapter 10.

Iron

Up to 25 percent of all women are iron deficient and should be aware of their risk of anemia. Anemia and iron deficiency are even more common in female athletes because of a combination of factors that include menstrual blood losses, iron loss in sweat, inadequate intakes of iron in normal diet, and the iron demands of adolescent growth spurts. Generally, women with anemia do not exhibit any symptoms, except in circumstances when the iron deficiency is severe. Early fatigue during exercise may be the only sign. The symptoms of severe anemia include extreme fatigue, irritability, and headaches. It is often difficult to evaluate the exact causes of anemia in the female athlete because of the multitude of factors that might cause the condition. A good rule of thumb is that when female athletes have hemoglobin levels in the low-to-normal range, they could probably benefit from daily iron supplements to provide for adequate reserves.

Calcium

If she is eating a well-balanced diet that provides enough calcium intake (1,000 milligrams per day), a normally menstruating sports-active woman

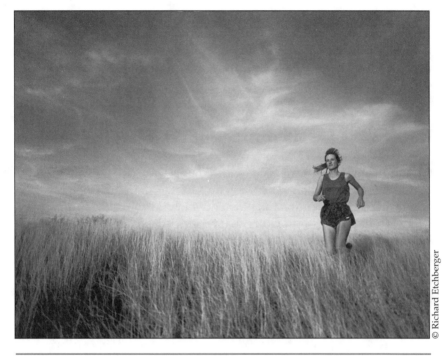

Female runners need to be vigilant about their nutritional intake.

need not consume additional calcium. However, nonmenstruating female athletes should consume 1,500 milligrams per day, and women who are experiencing irregular periods should take 1,200 milligrams per day. Supplemental calcium needs should ideally be met through diet. If this is not possible, supplements can provide adequate calcium intake. If supplements are used, calcium carbonate (40 percent elemental calcium) is the most concentrated form. Tums Ex antacid tablets are one of the least expensive and effective forms of calcium supplements (four cents a tablet).

Estrogen

Estrogen deficiency for any reason, whether before or after menopause, decreases bone density, predisposes the female athlete to stress fractures, and increases her susceptibility to complete fractures. Menstrual irregularities increase the risk of estrogen depletion. Bone mineral density among women with menstrual irregularities is lower than among women who are menstruating normally. Female athletes experiencing menstrual irregularities should seek help in returning to normal menstrual cycles, usually achieved by decreasing exercise and gaining weight.

If she fails to menstruate after 6 to 12 months, she should take estrogen supplements to preserve and possibly increase her bone mass.

If you have menstrual irregularity or have stopped having your periods altogether and you believe that poor eating habits are primarily to blame, you should have a nutrition checkup with a registered dietitian or a sports nutritionist. To find one, call the American Dietetic Association's National Center for Nutrition and Dietetics referral service at 800-366-1655.

Weight Control and Running

As part of the health boom, many people have taken up running primarily for weight control. The goal of most weight-control programs is to improve body composition, specifically the ratio of muscle to fat.

Exercise forms such as running are a more effective means of improving body composition than simple dieting. Dieting decreases metabolism, and since the dieter's body then needs fewer calories, less weight is lost. This commonly leads to the plateau phase, where weight loss slows or even stops. Often the dieter becomes frustrated and abandons the diet. During the plateau phase, the dieter must decrease calorie intake even further—a difficult proposition for even the most ardent dieter. Also, extreme calorie reduction may result in loss of lean body mass, primarily muscle.

By contrast, exercise increases the body's metabolism, and this effect persists for as long as 6 to 24 hours after exercising moderately for only 30 minutes. This results in increased fat loss compared to dieting.

It is important for those using exercise for weight control to remember that there may be no marked decrease in total weight. That is because muscle increases relative to fat, and muscle is heavier than fat. The scale may show the same weight as it did before the exercise program was started, even though a desirable change in the body is taking place. The looseness of clothes is a much better indication of positive weight change than the number on the bathroom scale. The ideal method of tracking body composition is through regular skin caliper tests. Many health clubs offer this service.

The most effective weight-control program combines calorie reduction with an increase in exercise. Energy expenditure must be greater than energy consumption. However, the dieter should lose no more than one or two pounds per week. The runner should modify the diet based on the food pyramid to be assured of receiving all the required nutrients.

Some runners may wish to increase their weight for appearance's sake. The aim of a weight-gain program should be to increase lean muscle

---

Proper and Improper Weight-Loss Programs

An estimated 60 to 70 million American adults and at least 10 million American teenagers are carrying around too much fat. Each year millions of these people embark upon weight-loss programs for aesthetic reasons, often without medical supervision.

Weight reduction is often recommended by physicians for medical reasons. It is well known that obesity is associated with a number of health-related problems, including overstraining the heart (added weight forces it to work harder), left ventricular dysfunction, high blood pressure, diabetes, kidney disease, gallbladder disease, respiratory dysfunction, joint diseases and gout, endometrial cancer, abnormal plasma lipid and lipoprotein concentrations, problems in receiving anesthetics during surgery, and impairment of work capacity.

Because so many people are affected by the problem of obesity, the American College of Sports Medicine (ACSM) has developed guidelines for safe and successful weight-loss programs.

In summary, a desirable weight-loss program

1. provides at least 1,200 calories per day for normal adults to meet their normal nutritional requirements;
2. includes foods acceptable to the dieter from the viewpoints of sociocultural background, usual habits, taste, cost, and ease in acquisition and preparation;
3. provides a negative calorie balance (not to exceed 500 to 1,000 calories per day less than recommended intake), resulting in gradual weight loss of no more than 2.2 pounds (1 kilogram) per week, without metabolic abnormalities;
4. includes the use of behavior modification to identify and eliminate dieting habits that contribute to improper nutrition;
5. includes an endurance exercise program of at least three sessions per week, 20 to 30 minutes per session, at a minimum of 60 percent of maximum heart rate; and
6. provides for new eating and physical activity habits that can be continued for life to maintain the achieved lower body weight.

mass. Muscle mass can only be increased by strength training supported by an increase in dietary intake based on the food pyramid, not by consuming any special food, vitamin, drug, or hormone.

Alcohol and the Runner

Many runners consume alcohol in social situations. Besides being a poor source of carbohydrates before exercise, alcohol is an unsatisfactory carbohydrate replacement after vigorous exercise. Alcohol consumption also compromises rehydration because it stimulates urination. Athletes seeking to replace lost carbohydrates should instead drink juices and other nonalcoholic fluids after exercise.

Alcohol is a popular postexercise libation among athletes. Consuming alcohol directly after exercise, however, carries its own problems. After vigorous exercise, athletes are generally dehydrated and undernourished. When they consume alcohol directly afterward, the alcohol enters the bloodstream more rapidly. Thus the effects of alcohol in dehydrated, undernourished athletes are more pronounced, and they should not operate automobiles in such situations.

Nutritionist Nancy Clark counsels against alcohol consumption, but makes the following recommendations for athletes who wish to have an alcoholic beverage after a workout: "Instead of consuming beer immediately after exercise, athletes should first quench their thirst with two or three 10- to 16-ounce glasses of water to replace sweat losses. Players should then eat some type of carbohydrate—such as fruit, a muffin, a bagel, or flavored yogurt (carbohydrates delay alcohol absorption better than protein or fat)—stretch, shower, and *then* relax at mealtime with a beer if desired."

Intelligent choices about drinking alcohol extend to nonathletic situations, too.

Alcohol is the most abused drug in the United States. There are approximately 10 million adult and 3.3 million 14- to 17-year-old problem drinkers. Alcohol is significantly involved in all types of accidents: motor vehicle, home, industrial, and recreational. Half of all traffic fatalities are alcohol related. Pathological conditions such as generalized skeletal myopathy, cardiomyopathy, pharyngeal and esophageal cancer, and brain damage are all associated with alcohol abuse. Its most prominent effect, though, is liver damage.

It is important for everyone to understand the effects of alcohol consumption on physical performance and the potential problems of long-term abuse.

According to the American College of Sports Medicine, a reasonable guideline to moderate, safe drinking for adults is to consume at one time no more than 0.5 ounces of pure alcohol per 50.7 pounds (23 kg) of body weight. This is the equivalent of three bottles of 4.5 percent beer, four one-ounce glasses of 14 percent wine, or three ounces of 50 percent whisky for a 150-pound (68 kilogram) man.

Index

U

Upper, shoe, 61
Urinary tract infections, 204-205
U.S. Department of Agriculture, 213-214

V

Vaginal infections, 204-205
Variable resistance machines, 38-39
Vegetables, 226-227
Verrucae, 109
Vitamins and minerals, 233

W

Warm-up, 17-19, 53
Warts, on feet, 109
Weight control, female runners, 241-243
Weights, free, 38, 39
Women. *See* Female runners
Workout structure, 17-20, 52-54

About the Authors

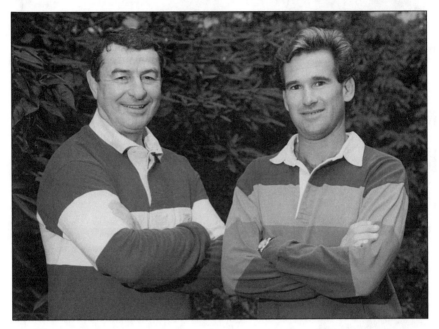

Lyle J. Micheli, who has been a clinical sports physician since 1973, is the director of the Division of Sports Medicine at Children's Hospital in Boston. A past president of the American College of Sports Medicine (ACSM), Dr. Micheli has served on the medical staff at the Boston Marathon every year since 1974—a longer span of continuous participation than any other living physician. Micheli is author of *The Sports Medicine Bible*, coauthor of *Sports for Life* and *Sportswise: An Essential Guide for Young Athletes, Parents, and Coaches,* and coeditor of four books, including the *Oxford Textbook of Sports Medicine.* He is also the author of many scientific articles on sports injuries in runners. In addition, he serves on the editorial and advisory boards of a number of sports medicine publications.

Dr. Micheli graduated from Harvard Medical School in 1966. He is a fellow of the ACSM and of the American Academy of Sports Medicine (formerly the American Orthopaedic Society for Sports Medicine). He is also chair of the Education Commission of the International Federation of Sports Medicine. During his professional career Dr. Micheli has received many honors, including the ACSM's Citation Award and the Krekor "Koko" Kassabian Award, which was presented by the Athletic Trainers of Massachusetts. A resident of Brookline, Massachusetts, Dr. Micheli enjoys cycling, skiing, and saltwater fishing.

Mark Jenkins is a freelance writer who has coauthored two health and fitness books. His first project with Dr. Micheli, *The Sports Medicine Bible,* was a Book-of-the-Month Club selection. In his leisure time Mark enjoys playing squash, soccer, and rugby.

Other Running Resources

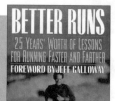
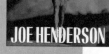

Joe Henderson

Foreword by Jeff Galloway

1996 • Paper • 264 pp • Item PHEN0866
ISBN 0-87322-866-9 • $14.95 ($19.95 Canadian)

Both an inspirational and instructional book that will boost motivation, performance, and enjoyment as a runner. Filled with anecdotes, insights, and advice on training, racing, and much, much more.

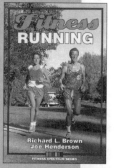

Richard L. Brown and Joe Henderson

1994 • Paper • 176 pp • Item PBRO0451
ISBN 0-87322-451-5 • $14.95 ($20.95 Canadian)

Contains helpful background information to get started in a running program, 60 color-coded workouts that vary in intensity and duration, and nine sample running programs.

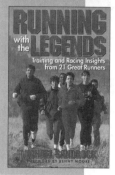

Michael Sandrock

Foreword by Kenny Moore

1996 • Paper • Approx 600 pp • Item PSAN0493
ISBN 0-87322-493-0 • $19.95 ($29.95 Canadian)

Details the development, training techniques, coaching, competitions, motives, and perspectives of 21 all-time great runners.

Human Kinetics
The Premier Publisher for Sports & Fitness
http://www.humankinetics.com

Prices are subject to change.

2335